SHEET PAN

COOKBOOK

DELICIOUS RECIPES FOR QUICK & EASY ONE-PAN MEALS

BY JOANNA MILLER

TABLE OF CONTENTS

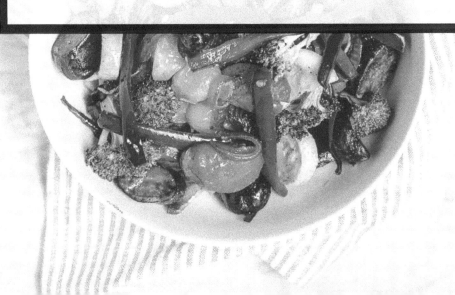

CHAPTER 1
INTRODUCTION

We all have one of those old baking sheets, you know the one I'm talking about. Don't try and deny it. It's tucked away in the dark section of your baking drawer. Judging you from the corner you shoved it into. You might have inherited it from your grandmother or purchased it on a whim after watching your favorite baking show.

There's no need to feel guilty and judged anymore! It's time to make your grandma proud or cash in on your spur-of-the-moment investment.

This might surprise you, but you can use that baking sheet for more than just cookies. You can make a full meal, plus dessert! I kid you not. This book is about to become the second-best purchase you've ever made! Your baking sheet being the first.

My fabulous Kitchen team has tried and tested all of the recipes. Allowing you the pleasure and ease of jumping right in with the confidence that these recipes will work. Just about everything can be perfectly cooked on your baking sheet, except for most pasta and rice variants. These unfortunately still need traditional cooking methods.

Your baking sheet will allow you the convenience of combining flavors on one mess-free sheet. No more keeping sides hot while the main meal is still cooking. No more transferring ingredients to ten different pots before it's ready. Have it all ready in one go.
Mingle with your guests while the dinner sorts itself out, your friends and family will think you've become a cooking genius overnight.

Developing these recipes together in our test kitchen and then trying them separately in our own homes, has given us a sense of what really matters for a great dinner. Great food, but more importantly, quality time spent with family and friends. In a very real way, the time saved during cooking was time well spent.

My deepest wish for the person holding this book is that you find the value that I did. Not just in cooking made easy, but in the true value of community that sharing a simple meal can bring.
Enjoy!

SHEET-PAN BASICS

These simple sheets of metal, are usually made of stainless steel or aluminum, and were invented for making cookies, buns and pastries. Yet we can do so much more with them.

Whether you call it a baking sheet, baking pan, oven tray, or just plain metal sheet, the definition remains the same. We use this piece of baking apparel for convenience and ease in the oven. You will usually find metal variations, but there are exceptions like glass,ceramic or some of the rare pottery kind. A unicorn if ever there was one, but they do exist.

They come in many shapes and sizes, yet the rectangle is the most popular and convenient choice with standard measurements that make the recipes in this book simple. You won't need to shop around for fancy, odd-shaped pans. The majority of the recipes use a 13 x 18-inch rimmed baking sheet. Although you can use any other shape or size that you may have on hand.

If you want to delve deeper into the magical world of baking sheets, here are a few sizes and their general uses, but there are no rules!

The larger sheet pans used by professionals or establishments are 18 x 26-inches.
The most common baking sheets that can be found in most homes are usually either small (quarter sheet pan) 12 1\2 x 8 1\2-inches. Or standard\medium (half sheet pans) 18 x 12-inches.
The standard measurements for the rim on most of these are 1 or 1 1\2-inches deep.

TIPS FOR COOKING WITH SHEET PANS

- To make your life as easy as possible. Spray your baking sheet with a baking spray or oil such as olive oil spray. You can Line your sheet with tin foil and coat the tin foil with spray to save on the life of your sheet. Use greaseproof paper instead of tin foil for fish and vegetables, this does not have to be sprayed.

- To save on time while using a single sheet pan, add the different foods at various times throughout your total cook time. Be meticulous in your prep and aim to slice, chop and dice food into roughly the same size pieces. This will ensure that everything will be done at the same time and you will not have uncooked bits in between. Making sure that the ingredients do not overlap which will also ensure even cooking.

- Keep your spatula and serving tongs at the ready for turning, stirring, and flipping food as well as removing the food from the sheet once it is done.

- Investing in a meat thermometer will ensure that your meat is always perfectly cooked to your preferences instead of guessing.

- You may notice that as a general rule with few exceptions, all meats and vegetables will need coating in some form of oil or sauce before baking. This will prevent them from burning and sticking.

- The maximum heat that your baking sheet can endure is 450°F, this may vary with special sheets, but this is the general temperature to go by.

- The rimmed baking sheet is of utmost importance if you don't want to spill all the juices and ingredients when you remove the sheet from the oven.

- Preheating may seem like an unnecessary step, but this will impact your cooking time, so make sure that you allow the general 15-30 minutes for your oven to properly preheat. Most ovens do have a convenient light to help you determine whether it's reached the desired temperature or not.

TIPS FOR CARING FOR SHEET PANS

- The best way to preserve your baking sheet is to wash it by hand. Baking sheets can be placed in the dishwasher but will eventually darken over time as a result.

- Allowing your baking sheet to cool completely before rinsing will prevent the metal from warping. Warped baking sheets will yield uneven cooking. If the food sticks to your sheet after cooling, fill your sheet with soapy water and allow it to soak for half an hour. Never use cold water in an attempt to cool your sheet faster. Patience is a virtue!

- If you don't want scratches on your pan, avoid using scourers or any abrasive sponges. Invest in a plastic scrub brush.

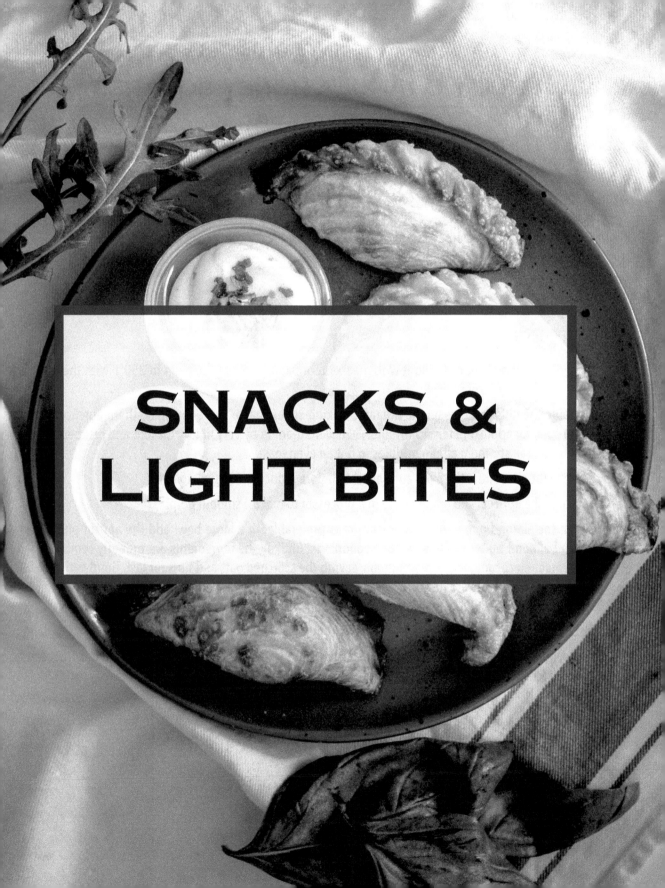

SNACKS & LIGHT BITES

FRUITY GRANOLA HONEY SQUARES

COOK TIME: 45 MINS | MAKES: 30 SQUARES

INGREDIENTS:

- 1 cup unsalted nuts of your choice
- 4 cups rolled oats
- ½ cup freshly squeezed orange juice
- 1 cup preserved apricots, diced
- ½ cup honey
- ¼ cup coconut oil
- ½ cup almond butter
- 1 cup puffed quinoa
- 1 cup grated coconut (Unsweetened is preferable)
- 1 tsp. lemon zest

DIRECTIONS:

1. Prepare a baking sheet by lining it with greaseproof paper. Preheat the oven to 350°F with the wire rack placed in the middle of the oven.

2. Combine the nuts and oats on the prepared baking sheet, making sure to spread them out. Scorch them in the oven for approximately 15 minutes, you want them to be very lightly toasted and just beginning to brown. You can stir them after 6 minutes to get an even toast.

3. Remove the sheet from the oven and set aside before reducing the oven to 300°F.

4. Combine the apricots and orange juice in a processor to make a smooth pulp.

5. Soften the almond butter, room temperature is preferable. In a large bowl add the apricot pulp, honey, oil, and almond butter. Using a wooden spoon, mix until all the ingredients are properly combined. Add the remaining coconut and puffed quinoa, saving the scorched oats and nuts for last. Gently mix until the remaining ingredients are just combined. Press the mixture securely into your sheet using your hands or the bottom of a measuring cup. Glass cups may work best.

6. Place the sheet in the oven for approximately 30 minutes or until the compacted mixture starts to darken.

7. Remove from the oven and allow to cool completely in the pan before cutting into squares. This can be done directly on the paper.

(Quick Tip) The squares can be stored in a cupboard, using a sealed container for up to two weeks. Leaving the parchment paper between the squares will prevent them from sticking together.

SPICY CHORIZO YAM BITES

COOK TIME: 20 MIN | MAKES: 48 BITES

INGREDIENTS:

- 1 lb. fresh chorizo with the casings removed
- 1 yam or ½ cup of baked, cooled, and mashed yam.
- 2¼ cups premade baking mix
- 8 oz. grated cheddar cheese
- ⅛ tsp. salt
- ⅛ tsp. ground cinnamon

- 2 tbsp. french mustard
- 6 tbsp. grape or plum jam
- pinch of rosemary

DIRECTIONS:

1. Prepare a baking sheet with a light layer of baking spray. Set the oven to preheat at 350°F.

2. In a bowl combine all the ingredients besides the mustard and jam. With your hands, roll the mixture into approximately 1½ inch balls and place them on the baking sheet, about an inch apart. You can also use a small ice cream scoop for more accurate measurements.

3. Bake for about 20 minutes or until the sausage is properly browned and sizzling.

4. With a fork in a small bowl, whisk the jam and mustard to make the sauce. If your jam is too thick you can always microwave it for a few seconds to make it easier to work with. The sauce can be poured over the bites or served on the side as an optional dip.

(Quick Tip) For quicker yam prep, you can cook the yam in the microwave for approximately 5 minutes on high. Poke or make small slices in the skin for easy removal. The yam can be turned after a few minutes. Allow to cool and then remove the skin before mashing. However, roasting the yam in the oven with a pinch of salt until soft will yield a better flavor.

CHEESY STUFFED ITALIAN MUSHROOMS

COOK TIME: 25-30 MINS | MAKES: 6-8 PORTIONS

INGREDIENTS:

- Olive oil
- 8 oz. of medium mushrooms
- 2 slices grain or brown bread
- 1/2 cup cream cheese
- 1/2 tsp. salt
- 1/2 tsp. garlic salt
- 1/2 tsp. Italian herb blend
- 2 tbsp. chopped fresh parsley

DIRECTIONS:

1. Begin preparations by preheating the oven to 350°F and lightly coating a pan with olive oil. You can use greaseproof paper to spread it evenly.

2. Rinse the mushrooms under fresh water and remove the stems. Allow the mushrooms to drain in a colander or pat dry with paper towels.

3. In a large bowl, combine the cream cheese and spices. Cube the bread before mixing it through the cream cheese and spices.

4. Place the mushrooms on the prepared pan and scoop even amounts of the cheese mixture onto each.

5. Decorate each mushroom with some parsley and bake for 20-35 minutes or until the mushrooms are soft and juicy.

SWISS CHEESE TART WITH MUSHROOMS

COOK TIME: 25 MINS | MAKES: 2-4 PORTIONS

INGREDIENTS:

- 1 packet puff pastry (roughly 8,5 oz.)
- flour for dusting
- 5 oz. grated swiss cheeses
- salt and pepper
- 4 1/2 tbsp. olive oil
- 2 spring onions, finely chopped
- ¼ lb. sliced mushrooms
- 1 large egg
- 1 tbsp. water
- ¼ cup (1¼ oz.) roughly chopped hazelnuts.
- ¾ lb. french green beans

DIRECTIONS:

1. To begin preparations, fit a baking tray with greaseproof paper and set the oven to preheat at 400°F.

2. Prepare a clean work surface by lightly dusting it with flour. Roll the pastry into an oblong shape that's roughly 12½-by-15-inch. After folding into thirds, gently move the dough to the pan and open. Be sure to leave enough room for the beans on the tray. Fold and pinch the edges of the pastry to create a 1 inch border all along the edge.

3. Spread the cheese evenly over the pastry. The edges should be visible with no cheese. Place the mushrooms and spring onions in a bowl. Sprinkle 3 tbsp of olive oil and season with salt and pepper to taste. Gently place the spiced mushrooms and spring onions over the grated cheese. In a small bowl, beat the egg with a fork and add 1 tbsp of water while beating. Using a brush, gently coat the pinched edges with the beaten egg. Place in the heated oven for 10 minutes.

4. Place the beans in a bowl and drizzle with 1 ½ tbsp olive oil and sprinkle with a pinch of salt and pepper. Move the seasoned beans to the tray beside the tart, fanning them out. Bake for another 10 minutes before sprinkling the crushed nuts over the beans and return the pan to the oven for an additional 5 minutes. The tart should be nicely browned and the beans should be soft when poked with a fork.

5. Remove the tray from the oven and allow to cool before slicing and serving with the French green beans on the side.

ROASTED CHICKPEAS WITH RANCH COATING

COOK TIME: 50 MINS | MAKES: ABOUT 2 CUPS

INGREDIENTS:

- 2 cans (19 oz. each) chickpeas, rinsed and drained
- 3 tbsp. olive oil
- 1/2 tsp. dried oregano
- 1 tsp. dried parsley
- 1/2 tsp. mustard powder
- 1/2 tsp. himalayan salt
- 1/2 tsp. onion powder
- 1/4 tsp. garlic powder
- pinch of ground cayenne pepper

DIRECTIONS:

1. Preheat the oven to 400°F and place the wire rack in the middle of the oven.

2. On the kitchen counter, place the chickpeas between two clean tea towels and gently roll them with the palm of your hands until all the shells are removed and the chickpeas are dry.

3. In a bowl, coat the chickpeas with the olive oil. Use a nonstick sheet or oven pan, fan the coated chickpeas out evenly. Place the pan or sheet in the oven and roast for approximately 50 minutes until the peas are evenly browned and burst open. Open the oven and move the peas around every 10 minutes.

4. While the Chickpeas are toasting, mix all the spices in a bowl.

5. When the Chickpeas are nicely roasted, coat them in the bowl of spices and add a pinch of salt and pepper. Set aside to cool completely before serving.

(Quick Tip) If the chickpeas start to lose their crispness, place them back in the oven and bake for a few minutes at 325°F until they are nice and toasted again. You can store them for a few days in a sealed container.

MINI SPINACH AND CHEESE PIES

COOK TIME: 10 MINS | MAKES: 15 SERVINGS

INGREDIENTS:

- 2 packets (1.9 Oz.) mini pastry shells
- 2 large eggs
- 10 oz. finely chopped spinach
- pinch of salt
- 4 oz. crumbled feta
- ½ tsp. oregano
- 1 tsp. crushed garlic

- ½ tsp. freshly ground black pepper
- juice from ½ lemon

Garnish:
- fresh dill
- black pepper
- salt

DIRECTIONS:

1. Set the oven at 375°F to preheat.

2. Arrange the shells on a lightly sprayed baking sheet and set aside.

3. In a bowl, beat the eggs and add the rest of the ingredients. Mixing to ensure everything is combined. Scoop the same amount of filling into each shell.

4. Place in the oven and bake for 10 minutes until the filling is set and the shells are nicely browned around the edges. Remove from the oven and allow to cool before garnishing with a sprinkling of black pepper and some chopped dill to give it an optional Mediterranean spin.

SPICY SHRIMP ON BAMBOO SKEWERS

COOK TIME: 8-10 MINS | MAKES: 8 SKEWERS

INGREDIENTS:

- olive oil
- 8 bamboo skewers
- 1 lb. cleaned, shelled, and deveined shrimp
- ½ lime, juiced
- 4 tbsp. butter
- 1 tsp. crushed garlic

- 3/4 tsp. southwest spice blend
- chopped fresh parsley

DIRECTIONS:

1. Set the oven to preheat at 350°F. Lightly coat a baking sheet with olive oil and set aside. Place your bamboo skewers near the baking sheet for easy access. Use paper towels to pat the shrimp dry.

2. In a saucepan over low heat, combine lime juice, spices, crushed garlic, and butter. Stir until the butter is melted, About 2 minutes, then remove the pan from the stove.

3. Divide the shrimp into batches and coat in the melted butter before spearing them onto the skewers. About 3 to 4 coated shrimp per skewer.

4. Arrange the skewers on your prepared baking sheet, making sure that they are not touching. Sprinkle the skewers with the chopped parsley. Bake for approximately 8-10 minutes or until the shrimp blush (turn a light shade of pink) and the tails start to curl. Monitor constantly as shrimp is easy to overcook and will become rubbery. A perfectly cooked shrimp will form a C when done.

5. Move the shrimp to a plate and serve.

CHILI CHICKEN BITES

COOK TIME: 30 MINS | MAKES: 12 PORTIONS

INGREDIENTS:

- 12 medium jalapeño chilies
- 1 cup cooked and shredded chicken
- 2 tbsp. finely chopped coriander leaves
- ¾ tsp. salt
- 1 tbsp. fresh lime juice
- 8 oz. soft cream cheese

- pinch of cayenne pepper
- 12 slices of thick bacon
- 24 wooden toothpicks

DIRECTIONS:

1. Set the oven to preheat at 400°F.

2. Prep your wire rack by lightly coating it with baking spray and use tin foil to cover your baking sheet.

3. Cut the chilies into long trips and use a teaspoon to scrape out the seeds and flesh on the inside.

4. With a wooden spoon, combine the shredded chicken, coriander, salt, lime juice, cream cheese, and cayenne pepper.

5. Spoon the mixture into the cleaned chili shells and smooth with the back of a teaspoon to fill all the gaps. Tightly wrap the bacon around each pepper and pin the bacon in place with toothpicks. Place your coated wire rack on the baking pan before arranging the peppers on the rack.

6. Roast in the oven for about 25 minutes or until the bacon starts to become crispy and the peppers are tender when poked with a fork.

7. Bring the oven up to broil and leave it for a few minutes until the bacon is completely crispy. Allow the poppers to stand for a few minutes after cooking.

CHEESY BAKED MUSHROOMS

COOK TIME: 8-10 MINS | MAKES: 8 SERVINGS

INGREDIENTS:

- 8 medium mushrooms
- 1 tbsp. cubed parma ham
- 6 tbsp. cream cheese
- olive oil
- pinch himalayan salt
- pinch of black pepper

DIRECTIONS:

1. Set the oven to preheat at 425°F.

2. Rinse the mushrooms under fresh water and remove all the dirt. Cut and discard the stems. Let the mushrooms drain in a colander or pat dry with paper towels.

3. Arrange the clean mushrooms on a lightly oiled baking sheet, leaving about an inch of space between each. Scoop even amounts of cheese into the mushroom caps. Use a teaspoon to press the cheese firmly into the caps before placing the Parma ham on top of the cheese. Sprinkle a bit of pepper and Himalayan salt on each mushroom.

4. Bake in your preheated oven for 8-10 minutes or until the mushrooms are tender when poked with a fork. Properly cooked mushrooms will begin to darken.

SPUNKY CHEESE SPUDS

COOK TIME: 2 HOURS | MAKES: 10 SERVINGS

INGREDIENTS:

- 1 lb. small potatoes
- 1 tbsp. olive oil
- 1½ tsp. himalayan salt
- 2 tsp. french mustard
- 2 tsp. finely chopped dill
- 2 tsp. finely chopped parsley

- 2 tbsp. preserved capers
- ½ cup sour cream
- 1 tsp. lemon zest
- 1 cup grated mozzarella

DIRECTIONS:

1. Set the oven to preheat at 350°F.

2. Rinse the potatoes under fresh water and pat dry with paper towels. Place the potatoes in a bowl and coat evenly with olive oil and salt. Arrange the potatoes on a lightly oiled baking pan and bake for about 40 minutes or until a knife can easily slide in and out. Move the potatoes to the kitchen counter and allow them to cool for about 15 minutes.

3. Half each potato with a knife. Using a teaspoon, gently hollow out the inside of each potato, taking care not to damage the skin. Keep the inside of the potatoes for later. Place the Potato cases in the oven and bake for an additional 10 minutes until the cases are dry. Remove from the oven and allow to cool completely for approximately 30 minutes.

4. With the scooped out potato from earlier in a large bowl, combine the remaining ingredients to form a mash. Divide the mash evenly between the potato cases and sprinkle with mozzarella. Return to the oven until the cheese has melted, about 5 minutes. Serve hot or allow them to cool for a tasty snack.

QUICK AND EASY CROISSANTS

COOK TIME: 10-12 MINS | MAKES: 12 SERVINGS

INGREDIENTS:

- ¾ cup warm water (100° to 110°f)
- 1 packet (¼ oz.) baker's yeast
- 2 tbsp. brown sugar
- 3 to 3 ½ cups bisquick
- coarse salt or sugar for sprinkling

DIRECTIONS:

1. In a small bowl, combine the warm water and yeast. Gently stir with a fork and set aside to bloom for about 5 minutes or until the mixture is foamy.

2. Using a wooden spoon in a large bowl, combine the sugar and 3 cups of Bisquick before gently adding the bloomed yeast to form a soft dough.

3. Place the dough on a lightly floured surface and gradually add the remaining Bisquick, working it through for about 10 minutes or until the dough is stretchy and no longer sticky to the touch.

4. Form a ball with the dough and roll it into a circle of about 12 inches. Using a knife or pizza cutter, slice the circle into 12 even pizza segments. Lightly coat a baking sheet with baking spray and set aside. Taking each individual segment, gently use your hands and roll them into a moon, starting at the bottom of the triangle and ending at the tip. Place the croissants on the prepared baking sheet with the points down. Cover the croissants on the sheet with a tea towel and allow to rise in a warm area for about an hour or until they are double their original size. A cold room with drafts will hinder the rising process.

5. While the croissants are rising, set the oven to preheat at 425°F. When they have properly risen, place them in the oven and bake for 10-12 minutes. The dough should be a crisp brown when done.

6. Depending on your preference of savory or sweet, you can sprinkle the warm croissants with either coarse salt or sugar.

MINI SWEET PEPPER TARTS

COOK TIME: 15 MINS | MAKES: 10 SERVINGS

INGREDIENTS:

- 1 packet of puff pastry
- 2 tbsp. mayonnaise
- 1\4 cup shredded mozzarella (1 oz.)
- 1 tsp. crushed garlic
- 3 or 4 mini sweet peppers, cut into rounds
- 8 baby tomatoes, sliced into rounds
- crushed thyme
- black pepper
- himalayan salt

DIRECTIONS:

1. Set the oven to preheat at 400°F. Use greaseproof paper to line a baking sheet.

2. After thawing your pastry, lightly flour your work surface and roll the pastry out to roughly 9x10 inches. Using a sharp knife, cut the dough into 20 even rectangles. Taking each piece, use your knife to draw a border right around, about 1\8 of an inch from the edges. Taking care not to cut all the way through. Using a skewer or toothpick, poke holes all over the inside of your pastry within the border, it does not have to be precise. Arrange your pastries on your baking sheet and allow them to rest for approximately 10 minutes in the fridge.

3. In a large bowl, combine the mayonnaise, mozzarella, and crushed garlic. On the rested dough pieces, spread a teaspoon of the mixture inside your cut border. Leaving the edges open. Arrange the sliced peppers and tomato on top of the cheese, about 2 slices of each per tart. Season with thyme, pepper, and salt.

4. Place the sheet in the oven and bake for about 15 minutes or until the pastry has puffed and browned.

CHICKEN SKEWERS IN PEANUT SAUCE

COOK TIME: 10-15 MINS | MAKES: 4 SERVINGS

INGREDIENTS:

- 1\2 tsp. cumin seeds
- 1 tsp. dried cilantro seeds
- 1 tsp. crushed garlic
- 1 tsp. brown sugar
- 1 tbsp. hoisin sauce
- 1 tbsp. soy sauce
- 1\2 tsp. ground curcuma
- 1\2 tsp. salt
- 2 tbsp. cashew oil

1 1\2 lb. cubed chicken breast

Sauce:
- 1\4 cup roasted peanuts
- 1\4 cup roasted cashew nuts (optional)
- 1\4 cup peanut butter
- 1\4 cup warm water
- 1\4 cup diced spring onions
- 1 tsp. crushed garlic
- 1\2 lime squeezed
- 1 tsp. fish sauce
- 1 tbsp. chili paste

- pinch of salt
- 1 tbsp. brown sugar

DIRECTIONS:

1. Set the oven to preheat on a broil. You want a piping hot oven for this recipe.

2. Using a dry skillet or wok over high heat, roast the cumin and cilantro seeds, tossing frequently for a few minutes until their flavors are evident. You will be able to smell when they are ready. Pour them from the pan into a grinder and crush into a coarse powder.

3. In a large bowl, whisk the roasted spice, crushed garlic, brown sugar, Hoisin sauce, soy sauce, Curcuma, salt, and cashew oil together. Mix the chicken cubes into the sauce and allow to soak for about 15 minutes.

4. Spear the chicken cubes onto your desired amount of skewers and arrange on a lightly sprayed baking sheet. Place the sheet in the oven for about 10 minutes. Flip the skewers after the first 5 minutes. The chicken should be properly cooked and browning on the edges.

5. In a separate bowl, combine and whisk all the ingredients for the sauce.

6. Arrange the skewers on a serving plate and pour the sauce over or serve on the side as an optional dip.

GORGONZOLA PIZZA WITH BBQ CHICKEN

COOK TIME: 10 MINS | MAKES: 6 SERVINGS

INGREDIENTS:

- 1 ready-made frozen pizza base. (8 oz.)
- olive oil
- 1\3 cup BBQ sauce
- 1\2 purple onion sliced into rings
- 1 1\2 cups diced roast chicken
- 1\2 cup sun-dried tomatoes
- 1 roughly chopped green pepper
- 1 cup crumbled gorgonzola cheese
- himalayan salt
- black pepper
- fresh basil leaves

DIRECTIONS:

1. Set the oven at 500°F to preheat.

2. Lightly spray a baking sheet with cooking spray. Place the pizza base on the sheet, brush with a thin layer of olive oil before spreading the BBQ sauce evenly over the oiled base. Take care to leave a 1-inch border around the edge.

3. Arrange the onions on the base and sprinkle with the chicken, tomatoes, green pepper, and cheese. Season with salt and pepper.

4. Place in the oven and bake for about 10 minutes or until the cheese has melted.

5. Remove from the oven and decorate with the optional Basil leaves before slicing and serving.

SPICY GERMAN PANCAKE WITH BACON

COOK TIME: 40 MINS | MAKES: 8 SERVINGS

INGREDIENTS:

- 1 lb. hickory smoked bacon, cut into squares
- 6 large eggs
- 1 1\2 cups full cream milk
- 1 1\2 cups flour
- ½ tsp. salt
- 3 tbsp. brown sugar
- 2 jalapeno chilies, chopped
- 1\2 lime, squeezed

- 1\4 tsp. raw honey
- 1 tbsp. olive oil
- pinch of himalayan salt
- pinch of ancho chili powder
- 1 cup freshly chopped rocket
- 1\2 cup whole kernel sweetcorn
- 1\2 cup sundried tomatoes
- 1 1\2 oz. queso cincho cheese, crumbled (1\3 cup)

DIRECTIONS:

1. Set the oven to preheat at 425°F.

2. Place the cubed bacon on a baking sheet, fanning it out. Place the sheet in the preheated oven and bake until the bacon is nice and crispy. About 20 minutes. Remove the sheet from the oven, leaving the bacon on the sheet, and set aside for later.

3. In a large bowl, with a whisk or hand mixer, beat the eggs and milk until light and fluffy. The more air you beat into your batter, the fluffier your pancakes will be. In a separate bowl, mix together all the flour, salt, and sugar. Gradually add your milk mixture to the flour while beating until completely smooth. Nobody likes lumpy pancakes! Beat for an extra few minutes to aerate the batter. Gently pour the batter over the bacon on the baking sheet. You can gently shake the tray to even it out. Spread the chilies over the batter before returning the sheet to the oven and baking for an additional 20 minutes or until your pancake bowl has puffed out.

4. While your pancake is baking, prepare your topping. In a large bowl, beat the lime, honey, olive oil, salt, and chili powder together. Add the rocket, sweetcorn, and tomatoes. Mix through with a wooden spoon until everything is coated.

5. When your pancake is ready, remove the sheet from the oven. Spread your coated ingredients over the pancake and sprinkle with cheese before serving.

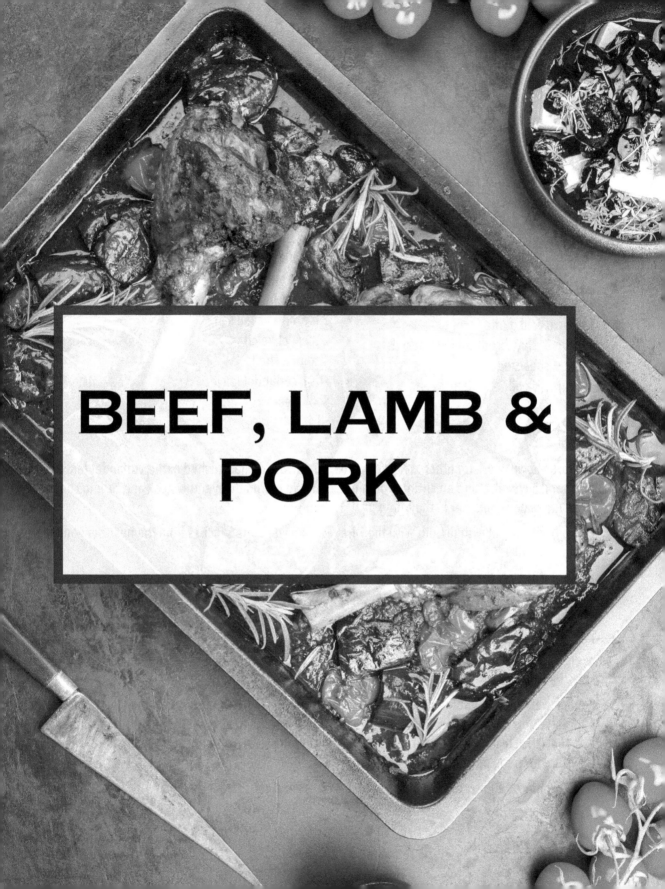

BEEF, LAMB & PORK

SPICY STEAK & YAM TACOS

COOK TIME: 35 MINS | MAKES: 6-8 SERVINGS

INGREDIENTS:

- 1-2 lb. fillet steak

Marinade:
- 4 tsp. himalayan salt
- 1 tbsp. ancho chili powder
- 1 tbsp. crushed jeera
- 1 tsp. crushed garlic
- 1\4 cup freshly diced coriander leaves
- 2 limes, squeezed
- 1\4 cup olive oil

Filling:
- 1\2 lb. mexican husk tomatoes, peeled
- 1 1\2 lb. yam, peeled and cubed. (3\4 inch cubes)
- 1 purple onion, diced
- 1 tsp. jeera
- 1 tsp. ancho chili powder
- 2 tsp. himalayan salt
- 2 tbsp. olive oil
- 4 tortilla shells
- Fresh coriander leaves
- Sour cream

DIRECTIONS:

1. In a large bowl, whisk together the salt, ancho chili powder, jeera, crushed garlic, coriander leaves, lime juice, and olive oil. Using an airtight container, pour the marinade over the steak and turn to coat evenly. Place the sealed container in the fridge for 1-12 hours.

2. Line a baking sheet with tin foil. With the wire rack placed about 6-inches from the heat, set your oven to preheat at 450°F.

3. Rinse and quarter the tomatoes. in a large bowl, combine the quartered tomatoes, yams, onion, jeera, chili powder, salt, and olive oil. Mix until everything is evenly coated. Spread the mixture over your baking sheet.

4. Place the baking sheet in the oven and bake for approximately 20 minutes. Remove the pan from the oven. Using a wooden spoon, create a well in the middle of your yam mixture and place the marinated steak in the center.

5. Set the oven to broil before returning the sheet to the oven for 12 minutes. Turn the steak after the first 6 minutes. You can use a fork to stir the yam mixture if it starts to burn. Remove the sheet from the oven and allow the steak to rest for 5 minutes before slicing the steak into strips across the grain. You can use the sauce from the pan to coat the meat.

6. Build your tacos and serve with fresh coriander leaves and sour cream on top.

MINI CASSEROLES WITH A TWIST

COOK TIME: 30 MINS | MAKES: 4 SERVINGS

INGREDIENTS:

- 1 1\4 lb. ground beef
- 1 small courgette, shredded
- 1\2 tsp. himalayan salt
- 1\2 tsp. black pepper
- 1\3 cup spiced bread crumbs
- 2 tbsp. french mustard

- 1 tbsp. olive oil
- 1\4 tsp. chili powder
- 1 tsp. chopped rosemary
- 3 small red apples, washed and sliced
- sliced chinese leeks for garnish

DIRECTIONS:

1. Set the oven to preheat at 425°F. Line a rimmed baking sheet with tin foil.

2. With a wooden spoon in a bowl, combine the meat, shredded courgette, salt, pepper and bread crumbs. With clean hands, mold your meat mixture into 4 tightly packed rectangles and place them separately on your prepared baking sheet. Use a brush to coat the tops with the French mustard.

3. In a separate bowl, whisk together olive oil, chili powder, and rosemary. Add the apple slices and coat evenly.

4. Place the coated apple slices around the meat on the tray. Move the sheet to the oven and bake for approximately 30 minutes, or until properly cooked.

5. Arrange the casseroles and apples on a serving plate and garnish with the Chinese leeks before serving.

MINI ITALIAN PIZZA PIES

COOK TIME: 45 MINS | MAKES: 4 SERVINGS

INGREDIENTS:

- 1\2 tsp. black pepper
- 1\2 tsp. himalayan salt
- 1\3 cup bread crumbs
- 1 tsp. italian herb blend
- 2 tsp. crushed garlic
- 1\2 small red onion, diced
- 8 oz. ground beef

- 1\2 cup tomato puree
- 1 lb. ready-made pizza dough
- 1\2 cup grated cheddar
- 1\2 cup grated mozzarella
- 1 tbsp. water
- 1 large egg

DIRECTIONS:

1. Prepare a baking sheet by lining it with tin foil. Set the oven to preheat at 400°F.

2. In a large bowl, with a wooden spoon, combine the pepper, salt, bread crumbs, Italian herb blend, crushed garlic, diced onion, and ground beef. With clean hands, roll the meat into 1-inch balls (16 balls) and place them on the prepared baking sheet. Not touching. Place the sheet in the oven and bake for approximately 12 - 15 minutes or until properly cooked. Be sure to keep an eye on the meatballs. Turn frequently to avoid burning.

3. When the meatballs are done, place them in a bowl with the tomato puree and set aside.

4. Turn down the heat in the oven to 375°F. Prepare a new baking sheet by lining it with tin foil and lightly coating the foil with baking spray.

5. On a lightly floured surface. Slice the dough into 4 even pieces. Using a rolling pin, roll each section into an 8-inch round. Place the meatballs in the center of each round, shifting them just to the side so that they are off-centered. 4 meatballs per round. Combine the two kinds of cheese in a bowl before sprinkling over the meatballs. Be sure to leave a 1-inch border around the edges. Fold the other half of the round over, closing the meatballs and cheese. Use a fork to seal the edges together by tightly pressing along the edges.

6. Arrange the mini pies on the prepared baking sheet and use a skewer to poke about 5 holes in each pie for the steam.

7. In a small bowl, beat the water and egg. Brush the top of each pie with your egg mixture before placing the sheet in the oven and baking for about 40 minutes or until nicely browned. Allow the pies to cool for 5 minutes before serving.

BUTTERY GORGONZOLA STEAK & VEGGIES

COOK TIME: 20 MINS | MAKES: 4 SERVINGS

INGREDIENTS:

- 2 cups rainbow heirloom tomatoes
- 1 1\2 lb. haricot verts
- 2 tbsp. olive oil
- 1 tsp. black pepper
- 1 1\2 tsp. himalayan salt
- 2 boneless, thick-cut steaks

- 1\2 tbsp. crumbled gorgonzola
- 3 tbsp. butter (room temperature)
- 1 tsp. chopped thyme
- 1 tsp. crushed garlic

DIRECTIONS:

1. Place the wire rack about 6-8 inches from the heat and set the oven to preheat on broil.

2. In a bowl, combine the cleaned tomatoes, Haricot verts, olive oil, 1 teaspoon salt, and 1\2 teaspoon pepper. Mix until evenly coated.

3. Place tomatoes and haricot verts on a baking sheet and broil in the oven for 5 minutes before removing the sheet from the oven.

4. Sprinkle the remaining salt and pepper on the steaks. Using a wooden spoon, make a well in the middle of the tomatoes and haricot verts, place the steaks in the center of the well. Return the sheet to the oven and broil for 2-4 minutes on each side. Adjusting the time to your desired rarity. Remove from the oven and allow to cool for 5 minutes.

5. In a bowl, whisk the gorgonzola, butter, thyme, and garlic. Arrange the steak, tomatoes, and haricot verts on a plate before pouring the cheese sauce over the steak.

SWEET & SOUR BEEF WITH BROCCOLI

COOK TIME: 25 MINS | MAKES: 4 SERVINGS

INGREDIENTS:

Marinade:
- 1\2 cup hoisin sauce
- 1 tsp. crushed garlic
- 2 spring onions, diced
- 1 tsp. grated ginger
- 1\2 tsp. sesame oil
- 2 tsp. mirin wine
- 2 tbsp. peanut oil

- 1\4 cup water
- 1\2 cup brown packed sugar
- 1\2 cup soy sauce

Beef and Broccoli:
- 4 lb. sliced beef
- 1 large head of broccoli
- cooked basmati rice for serving

DIRECTIONS:

1. In a pot over medium heat, whisk together all the ingredients for the marinade. Continuously stir until all the sugar granules have disappeared. Place the pot on a chopping board and leave to cool for 5 minutes.

2. Pour the marinade into an airtight container. Place the sliced beef in the marinade, and stir with a fork. Seal the container and chill for 30-45 minutes.

3. Cut the stems off the broccoli and clean with fresh water. Chop the broccoli into manageable portions.

4. Set the oven to preheat at 450°F. Lightly coat a sheet pan with sunflower oil before placing the pan in the oven to heat. Coat a wire rack with cooking spray.

5. When the oven has reached 450°F, carefully remove the sheet from the oven and place the wire rack on the sheet above the oil. Arrange the meat strips and broccoli on the rack and return the sheet to the oven for 10 minutes or until the meat is properly cooked, turning the meat and broccoli after the first 5 minutes. If you do not have enough room on the rack for all the meat and broccoli, you can place the cooked meat and broccoli in a bowl and cover with tin foil while you do another batch or two.

6. Take the remaining marinade and bring to a boil over a high heat for 30 seconds.

7. Dish the cooked rice, broccoli, and meat onto plates and pour the heated marinade over the rice.

CHEESY MINT HASLET

COOK TIME: 20 MINS | MAKES: 4 SERVINGS

INGREDIENTS:

- 1\2 cup crumbled feta
- 1 1\4 lb. ground beef
- Pinch of himalayan salt
- Pinch of black pepper
- 1\2 cup freshly chopped mint

- 6 small patty pans, 3 yellow and 3 green
- 1 green onion, finely chopped
- 1 tbsp. olive oil
- 1 cup green olives with the pips removed

DIRECTIONS:

1. Set the oven to preheat at 450°F. Line a baking sheet with tin foil.

2. Using a wooden spoon in a large bowl, combine the feta, beef, salt, pepper, and mint. Divide the meat into 4 equal portions and form them into tightly packed rectangles. Place the shaped meat onto the prepared baking sheet, leaving spaces between each for the vegetables.

3. In a separate bowl, combine the cleaned patty pans, chopped spring onion, olive oil, pinch of salt, and olives. Mix through until everything is properly combined. Arrange the coated vegetable on the sheet between the haslets and bake in the oven for about 20 minutes or until the haslet is completely cooked and browned. Remove from the oven and allow to rest for 5 minutes before serving.

HEARTY NACHO SALAD

COOK TIME: 25 MINS | MAKES: 6-8 SERVINGS

INGREDIENTS:

- vegetable oil
- 1 small onion, chopped
- 1 lb. ground beef
- 2 tsp. himalayan salt
- 1 oz. packet taco seasoning
- 14 oz. turtle beans
- 12 oz. frozen corn

- 1 head of iceberg lettuce, cleaned
- premixed salsa
- ranch sauce
- 1 cup crumbled cotija
- 1 cup grated cheddar
- corn chip of choice

DIRECTIONS:

1. Set the oven to preheat at 350°F. Coat a baking sheet with a thick layer of vegetable oil. The oil should flow over the sheet but not spill out.

2. In a bowl, combine the onions and ground beef, salt, and taco seasoning. Spread the mixture over half the pan and bake in the oven for about 20 minutes or until the meat is nicely browned. You can use a knife to cut through the meat and check to see that everything is evenly cooked. Turn the oven off. Place the beans, and corn on the sheet next to the meat and return to the cooling oven.

3. In your plates, layer the ingredients beginning with the lettuce, meat (You may have to break or cut the meat into manageable portions for layering), corn, beans, salsa, ranch, and cheese. Arrange the corn chips on the cheese or serve on the side.

FOUR SEASONS PORK BANGER SUBS

COOK TIME: 50 MINS| MAKES: 6 SERVINGS

INGREDIENTS:

- 2 large, red onions sliced
- 3 large sweet peppers, 1 green, 1 red, 1 yellow
- 1 cup mushrooms, sliced and cleaned
- 1 tsp. thyme
- 1 tsp. himalayan salt
- Pinch of black pepper

- 1 tbsp. olive oil
- 6 pork bangers
- 6 crisp sub rolls
- Butter

DIRECTIONS:

1. Set the oven to preheat at 375°F. Line a baking sheet with tin foil and lightly coat with baking spray.

2. Cut the peppers into strips and use a teaspoon to scrape out the seeds and inner flesh. In a bowl, combine the onions, pepper strips, mushrooms, thyme, salt, pepper, and olive oil. Stir with a wooden spoon to evenly coat. Place the coated vegetables on the baking sheet next to the bangers (They should not be touching) and poke each banger 3-4 times with a skewer.

3. Place the sheet in the oven and bake for 40 minutes. After 40 minutes, set the oven to broil and brown the sausages for 6-8 minutes, turning them after the first 4-5 minutes.

4. Open and butter the rolls generously before placing a banger in each and topping with the fried vegetables.

FULL SUNDAY LAMB-CHOP LUNCH

COOK TIME: 1 HOUR | MAKES: 4 SERVINGS

INGREDIENTS:

- Chops
- 4 tsp. crushed garlic
- 4 lamb-chops
- 4 tsp. freshly chopped rosemary
Marinade:
- 1\4 tsp. brown sugar
- 4 tbsp. olive oil
- 1\2 tsp. himalayan salt
- 1\2 tsp. black pepper

- 1 tsp. freshly chopped rosemary
- 1 tsp. crushed garlic
- 5 baby potatoes
- 4 medium carrots
- 1\4 pumpkin
- 4 tbsp. olive oil
- 1 tsp. salt
- 1 tsp. black pepper
- Cooked rice for serving

DIRECTIONS:

1. Place the lamb-chops on a cutting board. Make tiny slices with a sharp knife over each chop. Gently massage the garlic and rosemary into each chop (1 teaspoon of each per chop), flipping the chops after a few minutes and repeating the process on the other side. Set aside to rest.

2. In a small bowl, combine the sugar, olive oil, salt, pepper, rosemary, and garlic. Whisk with a fork. Use the marinade to once again massage the chops until evenly coated. Place the chops in a bowl and cover with tin foil. Set the covered bowl aside on the counter and allow to rest for 2 hours.

3. With the wire rack placed in the middle of the oven, set the oven to preheat at 450°F.

4. Clean, peel, and roughly cut all the vegetables. Place your vegetables in a bowl and coat with olive oil, salt, and pepper.

5. Coat a large baking sheet with a generous layer of olive oil and spread the vegetables over the sheet. Place in the oven and bake for 30 minutes, turning halfway through. Your vegetables are done when a fork or knife can easily be inserted.

6. Make a well in the middle of the vegetables and place the lamb chops in the center. Return the sheet to the oven and roast for about 30 minutes or until the chops have reached the desired rarity.

7. Remove from the oven and serve on a bed of rice.

SALISBURY LAMB STEAK WITH ZESTY PATE

COOK TIME: 50 MINS| MAKES: 6 SERVINGS

INGREDIENTS:

- 2 tsp. crushed garlic
- 2 1\2 tsp. ground jeera
- 1 1\2 tsp. ground cilantro seeds
- 3\4 tsp. paprika
- 1 tsp. himalayan salt
- 1\2 tsp. black pepper
- 1\4 lb. ground lamb

Pate
- 2 tbsp. olive oil
- 1 lb. baby artichokes
- 1\2 lemon, juiced
- Pinch of black pepper
- 1 tbsp. ground thyme
- 2 tbsp. orange zest, grated
- 1\2 cups brown olives with the pips removed

DIRECTIONS:

1. Line a baking sheet with greaseproof paper and set aside. Set the oven to preheat at 400°F.

2. Place the garlic, jeera, cilantro, paprika, salt, pepper, and ground lamb in a large bowl and mix with a wooden spoon until everything is combined. With clean hands, form the mixture into 12 patties and set aside.

3. In a small glass bowl, combine all the ingredients for the Pate and mix with a fork. Place in a food processor and pulse. Set aside.

4. To prepare the artichokes, fill a glass bowl with water and add the lemon juice. Peel the artichokes to reveal the heart and trim the stems. Quarter the artichoke hearts and place them in the lemon water when you aren't working with them. When you are done. Drain the artichokes in a colander, then generously coat them in olive oil, salt, and pepper, before arranging them on the prepared sheet and baking for 12-15 minutes.

5. Remove the sheet from the oven and use a spatula to move the artichoke hearts to the side, place the Salisbury steaks on the pan with a generous dollop of pate on each. Return the sheet to the oven and bake for an additional 12-15 minutes or until the steaks are cooked through. The artichokes should be tender when poked with a fork.

6. Plate and serve with the artichokes on the side.

SLOW ROASTED PISTACIA VERA LAMB

COOK TIME: 1 HOUR 30 MINS | MAKES: 6 SERVINGS

INGREDIENTS:

- 1 (4 lb.) boneless leg of lamb
- 2 tsp. ground cilantro seeds
- 3 tsp. crushed garlic
- 1 tsp. salt
- 1 tsp. black pepper
- 1 lb. radish, cleaned, peeled and, quartered
- 1 lb. carrots, cleaned, peeled and, quartered
- 2 spring onions, chopped
- 2 tbsp. olive oil

- 1\4 tsp. himalayan salt
- 2 tsp. lemon zest
- 1\2 cup chopped parsley
- 1\2 cup chopped mint leaves
- 1\2 cup roasted and salted pistacia vera nuts

DIRECTIONS:

1. Set the oven to preheat at 325°F.

2. Place the lamb on a chopping board. Combine the cilantro, garlic, salt, and pepper in a small bowl. Whisk with a fork. Use the spice mixture to gently massage the lamb all over, until all the spice is mixed in. Roll the lamb into a barrel and fasten at both ends using butcher's twine, add twine at 2-inch intervals. This will hold the meat together.

3. Line a baking sheet with tin foil and place a wire rack over the sheet. Place the lamb on the rack and roast in the oven for 1 hour. After an hour, reduce the heat to 475°F.

4. In a large bowl, coat the vegetables with olive oil and salt. Arrange the vegetables on a lightly oiled baking sheet and roast in the oven with the lamb for 30 minutes or until the vegetables are tender. The lamb should be cooked all the way through.

5. While the lamb and vegetables are baking. Place the lemon zest, parsley, mint, and Pistacia vera on a chopping board and roughly chop with a sharp carving knife. Place the combined spices in a bowl.

6. Arrange the cut lamb and vegetables on the plates and sprinkle with the chopped spices before serving.

MOROCCAN RAITA LAMB SKEWERS

COOK TIME: 20 MINS | MAKES: 4 SERVINGS

INGREDIENTS:

- 1\2 tsp. cayenne pepper
- 1\2 tsp. ground ginger
- 1\2 tsp. himalayan salt
- 1\2 tsp. black pepper
- 1 tbsp. ground jeera
- 1 tsp. cardamom
- 2 cloves of garlic, chopped
- 2 tbsp. olive oil
- 12 lamb chops

Raita
- 2 tbsp. mint, chopped

- 1 small cucumber grated
- 1 lemon juiced
- 1 1\2 cups unsweetened yogurt
- 3\4 ground jeera
- 1\2 tsp. lemon zest
- 1 small courgette
- 1 sweet pepper
- 1 medium patty pan
- 1\2 red onion
- 4 tbsp. olive oil
- 1\2 tbsp. balsamic vinegar
- 4 pieces naan bread

DIRECTIONS:

1. Combine the cayenne pepper, ginger, salt, pepper jeera, cardamon, and olive oil in a small bowl. Place the chops on a wooden board and use the mixed spices to massage the chops and coat evenly. Cover with foil and allow to rest for 30 minutes on the counter.

2. Line a baking sheet with tin foil and set the oven to preheat at 375°F. If you are using wooden skewers, allow them to soak in warm water for at least half an hour before using.

3. Mix the mint, cucumber, lemon juice, yogurt, jeera, and lemon zest in a small bowl. Season with a pinch of salt and pepper. Put aside for later.

4. Wash, peel and cut all of the vegetables into roughly the same size squares. Place in a large bowl and coat with olive oil, vinegar and season with salt and pepper. On a wooden board, cut the lamb onto rough cubes. Build your skewers by alternating the vegetables and meat. Arrange the skewers on the prepared sheet and bake in the oven for 20 minutes or until the lamb is cooked and the vegetables are tender.

5. Brush the Naan on both sides with olive oil and place them on the outer corners of the sheet for the last two minutes of the skewers baking.

6. Arrange the skewers and toasted Naan on a plate and skewers with the raita on the side.

CHEESY CRUMBED PORK CHOPS

COOK TIME: 30 MINS | MAKES: 4 SERVINGS

INGREDIENTS:

Vegetables
- 1 pepper squash
- 3 lb. baby potatoes
- 2 tbsp. olive oil
- 1 tsp. crushed garlic
- 1\2 tsp. salt
- 1\2 tsp. black pepper

Crumbed pork chops
- 1\2 cup grated parmesan

- 1 cup bread crumbs
- 2 tbsp. corn flour
- 4 boneless pork chops
- 1\4 cup mayonnaise

Sauce
- 1 tbsp. honey
- 2 tbsp. whipped cream
- 2 tbsp. english mustard
- 1\4 cup sour cream with chives

DIRECTIONS:

1. Set the oven to preheat at 425°F and place both the wire racks in the middle of the oven.

2. Clean, peel and cut all of the vegetables into small squares (1\2 inch.) Place the chopped vegetables in a large bowl and coat with the garlic, olive oil, salt, and pepper. Arrange on a lightly sprayed baking sheet and roast on the lower rack for 10 minutes before turning with a spatula.

3. In a small bowl, whisk together the parmesan, bread crumbs, and corn flour with a fork. Place the pork chops on a wooden board and season with salt and pepper. Use a basting brush to coat both sides of the chops with the mayonnaise. Sprinkle the crumb mixture onto a plate and coat the pork chops evenly. Arrange the coated pork chops on a lightly sprayed baking sheet and bake above the vegetables for 15 minutes. Turn the oven up to broil after 15 minutes and brown the coating evenly on both sides. 2 1\2 minutes each.

4. In a small bowl with a fork, whisk together the honey, whipped cream, sour cream, and mustard.

5. Plate the pork chops and vegetables. Pour the sauce over the chops and serve.

CANTONESE FILLET MIGNON

COOK TIME: 25 MINS | MAKES: 4 SERVINGS

INGREDIENTS:

- 2 tbsp. brown sugar
- 2 tsp. crushed garlic
- 1 tsp. chili sauce
- 3 tbsp. soy sauce
- 1\4 cup sunflower oil
- 1\2 tsp. chili flakes
- 1\3 cup hoisin sauce
- 2 pork fillets

- 3 lb. haricot verts
- 2 medium yams
- 2 tbsp. sunflower oil

DIRECTIONS:

1. Combine the brown sugar, crushed garlic, chili sauce, soy sauce, sunflower oil, chili flakes, and hoisin sauce in a glass bowl and whisk. Coat the filets with the marinade and place in an airtight container. Chill for 8-12 hours.

2. Set the oven to preheat at 425°F and place the rack in the middle of the oven.

3. Wash, peel, and quarter the yams. Trim the stems off the haricot verts. Place the cleaned and cut vegetables in a large bowl and season with oil, salt, and pepper. Place the seasoned vegetables on a lightly oiled baking sheet and bake for 10 minutes or until a knife can be easily inserted into the yams.

4. Remove the sheet from the oven and turn the vegetables with a spatula. Make a well in the middle of the vegetables and place the fillets in the center, pouring all the marinade from the container onto the meat. Return the sheet to the oven and bake for 15 minutes or until the chops are completely cooked.

5. Remove the sheet from the oven and cover with tin foil, allowing the meat to rest for 5 minutes before slicing and serving.

SPICY PORK AND APPLE BAKE

COOK TIME: 30 MINS | MAKES: 4 SERVINGS

INGREDIENTS:

- 3 tbsp. plus 2 tsp. olive oil
- 4 pork chops
- 1\2 tsp. black pepper
- 1 tsp. himalayan salt
- 3 tbsp. packed brown sugar
- 2 tsp. crushed rosemary
- 1\8 tsp. ground cinnamon
- 1 tsp. garlic salt
- 1 tsp. paprika
- 1 tsp. chili flakes
- 1 tbsp. honey
- 3 tbsp. apple cider vinegar
- 1 lb. brussel sprouts, cleaned and trimmed
- 1 large red apple, cored and sliced (1\2 inch wedges)

DIRECTIONS:

1. Set the oven to preheat at 425°F.

2. Place the pork chops on a wooden chopping board and massage each chop with 1\2 teaspoon of olive oil and set aside. In a small bowl, combine 1\4 teaspoon pepper, 1\2 teaspoon salt, 1 tablespoon sugar, 1 teaspoon rosemary, cinnamon, garlic salt, paprika, chili flakes, and honey. Rub the mixed spices into the chops.

3. In a small glass bowl, whisk together the apple cider vinegar, 2 tablespoons of brown sugar, and the remaining spices, gradually drizzling in the 3 tablespoons of olive oil until everything is blended.

4. In a large bowl, coat the apple slices and sprouts with 1\4 cup of the apple cider mixture.

5. Line a baking sheet with tin foil and spray with baking spray. With the pork chops in the center of the sheet, arrange the coated apple slices and sprouts around the chops. Place the sheet in the oven and bake for 12 minutes before turning the chops and baking for an additional 12 minutes or until the chops are properly cooked.

6. Remove the sheet from the oven. Place the pork chops in a covered bowl and set aside. Fan out the apples and sprouts before returning to the oven on broil for about 5 minutes until everything has crisped. Remove from the oven and combine with the remaining apple cider mixture. Stir to evenly coat.

7. Plate the pork chops and serve the apples and sprouts on the side.

BAKED PORK RISONI

COOK TIME: 40 MINS | MAKES: 6 SERVINGS

INGREDIENTS:

- 2 lb. pork fillet
- 2 lemons, thinly sliced
- 1\2 tsp. himalayan salt
- 1\2 tsp. black pepper
- 4 tsp. olive oil
- 2 garlic cloves, chopped
- 1\2 onion, chopped
- 2 bunches of spinach, cleaned and chopped
- 1 lb. risoni, cooked

DIRECTIONS:

1. Use tin foil to line a baking sheet and set the oven to preheat at 450°F.

2. In a large bowl, combine the fillets, lemon slices, salt, pepper, and olive oil. Mix until the fillets are properly coated.

3. Arrange the fillets and lemon slices on the prepared baking sheet and bake in the oven for 30 minutes or until the fillets are properly cooked.

4. Heat 2 teaspoons of olive oil in a pan and add the garlic and onions. When the garlic and onions are tender, add the spinach and allow to cook for 7 minutes with the lid on the pot.

5. When the spinach is cooked, combine it with the cooked pork and lemons. Serve on a bed of cooked Risoni.

SHREDDED PORK BUNS

COOK TIME: 15 MINS | MAKES: 8 SERVINGS

INGREDIENTS:

- 1\2 cup water
- 8 pre-packed Chinese buns
- 1 tbsp. olive oil
- 1\2 tsp. salt
- 1\2 tsp. pepper
- 1 lb. pulled pork
- 1 1\2 tbsp. plain rice vinegar
- 1 1\2 tbsp. ponzu sauce
- 3 tbsp. tangy mayonnaise

- 1\4 cup gochujang sauce
- 1 cup cucumber, sliced
- 1\2 cup shredded carrots
- 1\4 cup red onions, diced and cooked
- 1\4 cup coriander leaves, chopped
- 1\2 lime

DIRECTIONS:

1. Set the oven to preheat at 475°F. Arrange 2 racks on the second positions from the top and the bottom. Spray a wire rack with baking spray and place it over a rimmed baking sheet. Pour the water into the sheet. Measure and spray a piece of tin foil to cover the sprayed rack. It needs to be bigger than the rack so that it can tent the buns. Arrange the buns on the rack and cover them with the foil. Sprayed side down. Pinch the foil over the edges of the rack to form a secure tent.

2. In a large bowl, combine and toss the olive oil, salt, pepper, and pork until evenly coated. Lightly spray a tin foil-lined baking sheet. Arrange the pork on the sheet and place it on the top rack in the oven, with the buns on the bottom rack. Bake for 10 minutes before increasing the oven to broil and baking for another 5 minutes until the pork is nice and crispy.

3. In a large bowl, whisk together the rice vinegar, ponzu sauce, mayonnaise, and gochujang sauce. Add the cooked pork and mix until evenly coated. Divide the mixture evenly between the buns.

4. In a separate bowl, combine the cucumber, carrots, onions, coriander leaves, sprinkle with the lime juice, and a pinch of salt and pepper. Top the buns with the fresh mixture and serve.

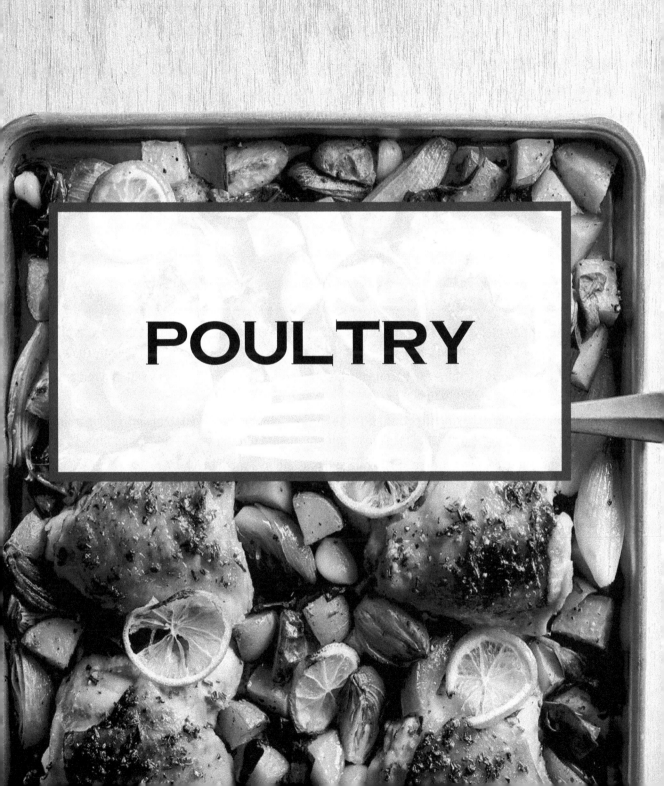

POULTRY

ROASTED CHICKEN WITH BACON BITS

COOK TIME: 50 MINS | MAKES: 4 SERVINGS

INGREDIENTS:

- 2 tsp. crushed garlic
- 1 tbsp. french mustard
- 4 tbsp. olive oil
- 1 tsp. himalayan salt
- 1\2 tsp. black pepper
- 2 lb. chicken (any cut of your choice)
- 1 1\2 lb. potatoes, cleaned, peeled, and quartered
- 3 slices thick bacon, cubed

- 10 oz. mushrooms, cleaned and sliced
- 2 onions, sliced
- 2 spring onions, cleaned and sliced
- 1 cup heavy cream
- 2 tbsp. english mustard
- 2 tsp. thyme
- 6 fresh thyme sprigs for garnish
- Cooked rice

DIRECTIONS:

1. Set the oven to preheat at 425°F. In a large bowl, combine the garlic, mustard, 2 tablespoons olive oil, 1\2 teaspoon salt, 1\4 teaspoon pepper, chicken, and potatoes. Mix until everything is evenly coated.

2. In a separate bowl, combine the bacon, mushrooms, onions, and spring onions with the remaining olive oil, salt, and pepper. Stir to coat.

3. On a lightly sprayed baking sheet, arrange the chicken, potatoes, and vegetable mixture in a single layer. Place the sheet in the oven and bake for 15 minutes before turning and baking for another 15 minutes.

4. For the coating, combine the cream, thyme, and mustard in a small bowl.

5. After 30 minutes, remove the chicken from the oven and coat evenly with the cream mixture. You can drizzle any remaining cream over the potatoes and vegetables. Return the sheet to the oven and bake for 20 minutes or until the chicken is nicely roasted and cooked all the way through.

6. Garnish with the fresh thyme and serve on a bed of rice.

ROASTED CHIMICHURRI LIME CHICKEN

COOK TIME: 45 MINS | MAKES: 6 SERVINGS

INGREDIENTS:

- 1\2 tsp. crushed red pepper flakes
- 1 1\2 tsp. himalayan salt
- 1\2 cup red wine vinegar
- 1\4 cup olive oil
- 1\3 cup coriander leaves, chopped
- 1\2 cup onions, chopped
- 1\2 lime, squeezed

- 4 lb. quarters chicken
- 1 lb. potatoes, cleaned, peeled, and quartered
- 1 tbsp. paprika
- 2 spring onions, chopped
- Fresh coriander for garnish

DIRECTIONS:

1. Line a baking sheet with tin foil and coat with olive oil. Set the oven to preheat at 425°F.

2. In a large bowl, combine the pepper flakes, 1 teaspoon salt, 2 tablespoons vinegar, 2 tablespoons olive oil, coriander leaves, onions, and lime juice. Remove the skin from the chicken and set aside. Use the lime mixture to evenly massage the chicken before replacing the skin. You can use 3 or 4 toothpicks to hold the skin in place.

3. In a separate bowl, combine the potatoes with 1 tablespoon of olive oil, spring onions, remaining salt, and paprika. Mix until evenly coated.

4. Arrange the chicken and potatoes on the prepared baking sheet and bake for 35 minutes or until the chicken is properly cooked. Remove the chicken onto a wooden board and let it rest for 5 minutes. Meanwhile, return the vegetables to the oven and broil for 5 minutes or until they are crispy.

5. Plate the chicken and potatoes before topping with the remaining vinegar and garnishing with fresh coriander.

OLIVE STUFFED SALAMI CHICKEN

COOK TIME: 30 MINS | MAKES: 4 SERVINGS

INGREDIENTS:

- 4 chicken breasts, thinly sliced
- 1 lb. carrots, sliced
- 1 lb. cauliflower (slice about the same size as the carrots)
- 1\2 tsp. pepper
- 1\2 tsp. salt
- 2 tbsp. olive oil
- 1 tbsp. balsamic vinegar
- 2 tbsp. olive oil

- 1\2 tsp. cayenne pepper
- 1\2 cup celery leaves
- 1 tsp. crushed origanum
- 1 cup green olives, pitted and chopped
- 1\2 cup chopped and roasted red sweet peppers
- 1\2 cup onions, chopped
- 4 slices salami
- 4 slices provolone

DIRECTIONS:

1. Wrap each breast in cling wrap and tenderize on a wooden board by gently hammering both sides with a cooking mallet.

2. In a large bowl, combine the carrots, cauliflower, pepper, salt, and olive oil. Stir until everything is evenly coated. Line a baking sheet with a thin layer of olive oil before arranging the vegetables on the sheet and baking for 10 minutes.

3. Combine the vinegar, 2 tbsp. Olive oil, cayenne pepper, celery leaves, oreganum, olives, peppers, and onions in a bowl and mix until evenly coated.

4. To make the wrapped chicken, place a tenderized chicken breast on a slice of salami. Place a slice of cheese neatly in the center of the breast and top with a teaspoon of the olive mixture. Gently wrap the chicken and salami into a cylinder and pin in place with 2 or more wooden skewers. Set the remaining olive mixture aside for later.

5. After 10 minutes, remove the vegetables from the oven and use a spatula turn. Make a well in the middle of the vegetables and place the chicken in the center. Return the sheet to the oven and bake for an additional 15 to 20 minutes or until the chicken is properly cooked and the vegetables are nice and crispy.

6. Plate the rolled-up chicken after removing the skewers and garnish with the remaining olive mixture.

SPICY PAPRIKA BREADED CHICKEN

COOK TIME: 20 MINS | MAKES: 4 SERVINGS

INGREDIENTS:

- 1 large egg
- 3 tbsp. whole grain mustard
- 1\2 tsp. smoked paprika
- Pinch of salt
- Pinch of pepper
- 4 chicken breasts
- 1 cup bread crumbs

- 2 tbsp. corn flour
- 2 tbsp. olive oil
- 1 lb. carrots, cut into strips

DIRECTIONS:

1. Preheat the oven to 450°F. Prepare two baking sheets by coating them with a light layer of baking spray.

2. In a large bowl, beat the egg, mustard, paprika, salt, and pepper. In a separate bowl, combine the bread-crumbs and corn flour. Coat the chicken breasts in the egg mixture before coating them with the bread crumbs. Arrange the coated breasts on one of the baking sheets.

3. Toss the carrots in a bowl with the olive oil and a pinch of salt and pepper before fanning them out on the second sheet.

4. Place both sheets in the oven and bake for 20 minutes or until the chicken is properly cooked and the carrots are fork-tender. Serve as desired.

SPICY CHICKEN MARAQ

COOK TIME: 25 MINS | MAKES: 4 SERVINGS

INGREDIENTS:

- 4 lb. spicy lamb sausage, sliced
- 4 lb. chicken breasts, cubed
- 2 tsp. crushed garlic
- 2 onions, chopped
- 1 tsp. curry powder
- 1\4 tsp. crushed anise seeds
- 3 tbsp. olive oil
- 2 courgettes, thinly sliced
- 1\4 cup coriander leaves
- 1\4 cup preserved apricots, diced
- Lemon wedges for serving

DIRECTIONS:

1. Line a baking sheet with greaseproof paper and preheat the oven to 425°F, with the rack in the middle of the oven.

2. In a large bowl, toss together the sausage, chicken, garlic, onions, curry powder, anise, and olive oil until evenly coated. Spread the mixture out onto the prepared baking sheet and bake for 12 1\2 minutes before turning and baking for an additional 12 1\2 minutes.

3. In a bowl, coat the courgettes and dried apricots with the olive oil. Remove the pan from the oven and add the vegetables before returning to the oven and baking for 5 minutes or until the chicken is properly cooked and the vegetables are tender and crisp.

4. Plate the chicken and vegetables, season with salt, pepper, and the coriander leaves before serving with the lemon wedges on the side.

ROASTED HONEY & MUSTARD CHICKEN

COOK TIME: 45 MINS | MAKES: 4 SERVINGS

INGREDIENTS:

- 4 chicken quarters
- 3 tbsp. olive oil
- 1 1\2 tsp. black pepper
- 1 3\4 tsp. himalayan salt
- 2 garlic cloves, finely chopped
- 1 purple onion, cut into wedges
- 1 lb. brussel sprouts, cleaned, trimmed, and halved

- 3 cups cubed pumpkin
- 1\2 tsp. french mustard
- 1 tbsp. raw honey
- 2 tbsp. rosemary, chopped

DIRECTIONS:

1. Set the oven to preheat at 425°F. Line a baking sheet with baking spray and place in the oven for 5 minutes to heat while you prepare the chicken.

2. Use a basting brush to evenly coat the chicken with 1 tablespoon of olive oil and season with 3\4 teaspoons each of the salt and pepper. Place the chicken on the heated baking sheet with the skin down and bake for 10 minutes.

3. In a large bowl, combine the pumpkin, sprouts, onions, garlic, 1 1\2 tablespoons olive oil, and the remaining salt and pepper. Mix until evenly coated.

4. In a small bowl, whisk together the remaining olive oil, mustard, and honey.

5. Remove the chicken from the pan and place the coated vegetables on the pan, fanning them out. Arrange the chicken on top of the vegetables and brush the chicken with the honey and mustard mixture.

6. Return the sheet to the oven for 15 minutes. Take the sheet out of the oven and baste the chicken with the pan juice before sprinkling it with the rosemary and baking for an additional 20 minutes or until the chicken is properly cooked.

(Quick Tip) If the chicken is browning too quickly, you can use tin foil to cover the chicken while it bakes.

SPICY CHICKEN WITH BACON SPINACH

COOK TIME: 40 MINS | MAKES: 4-6 SERVINGS

INGREDIENTS:

- 1 tbsp. salt
- 1 tsp. black pepper
- 1\2 tsp. paprika
- 1 tsp. onion powder
- 3 tsp. crushed garlic
- 1 tsp. cayenne pepper
- 1\2 cup hot sauce (whichever is your favorite)
- 1\2 cup apple cider vinegar
- 1 cup plain yogurt

- 1 tsp. chili flakes
- 3 lb. chicken cuts of your choice.
- 1 lb. yams, cleaned, peeled, and cut into small cubes
- 3 tbsp. olive oil
- 2 slices thick-cut bacon, cubed
- 1 onion, sliced
- 3 cups spinach, cleaned and finely chopped
- 1 cup crumbled feta

DIRECTIONS:

1. In a large bowl, whisk together the salt, pepper, paprika, onion powder, garlic, cayenne pepper, hot sauce, apple cider vinegar, yogurt, and chili flakes. Place the chicken cuts in the sauce, mix to evenly coat. Allow the chicken to marinate for at least 12-24 hours in the fridge in an airtight container.

2. Set the oven to preheat at 425°F.

3. Combine the cubed yams with 1 tablespoon of olive oil and season with salt and pepper. Mix until evenly coated.

4. On a lightly greased baking sheet, arrange the marinated chicken and coated yams. You want to shake off any excess marinade before placing the chicken on the sheet. Place the sheet in the oven and bake for 20 minutes.

5. In your bowl from earlier, combine the bacon, onions, spinach, 2 tablespoons of olive oil, and season with a pinch of salt and pepper. Remove the sheet from the oven and flip the chicken and yams, pushing them to the side. Add the spinach to the sheet and bake for an additional 20 minutes or until the chicken is properly cooked and the spinach is done.

JAMAICAN ROAST CHICKEN

COOK TIME: 1 HOUR 15 MINS | MAKES: 4 SERVINGS

INGREDIENTS:

- 1\4 tsp. black pepper
- 1\2 tsp. salt
- 1\4 tsp. ground allspice
- 1 tbsp. brown packed sugar
- 1 1\2 tbsp. soy sauce
- 1 1\2 tbsp. freshly squeezed lime juice
- 2 tbsp. olive oil

- 2 tbsp. melted butter
- 1 tbsp. sliced chilies
- 1 sprig of fresh rosemary
- 2 spring onions, chopped
- 1 whole chicken

DIRECTIONS:

1. Set the oven to preheat at 425°F. Line a baking sheet with tin foil and place a wire rack over the foil.

2. In a food mixer, pulse the pepper, salt, allspice, sugar, soy sauce, lime juice, olive oil, butter, chilies, rosemary, and onions to form a creamy paste.

3. On a wooden board, gently massage the skin away from the chicken, taking care not to tear the skin. Spoon the paste between the skin and the chicken, massaging it in as you go. Use the leftover paste as a baste rub all over the outside of the chicken skin. Use butcher's twine to tie the drum sticks together and fasten the wings to the sides.

4. Place the chicken on the prepared rack and roast in the oven for 1 hour. After an hour, reduce the heat to 375°F and roast for an additional 15 minutes or until the chicken is properly cooked and the skin is crispy.

5. Remove from the oven, carve and serve.

TANGY ROAST CHICKEN

COOK TIME: 35 MINS | MAKES: 4-6 SERVINGS

INGREDIENTS:

- 1 tbsp. brown sugar
- 1 tbsp. mirin
- 1 tbsp. rice vinegar
- 1\4 cup white miso paste
- 1 spring onion, finely chopped
- 6 chicken drumsticks or thighs
- 1\4 tsp. himalayan salt
- 1\4 tsp. black pepper
- 2 spring onions, finely chopped
- 3 tbsp. canola oil
- 10 brussel sprouts, cleaned, peeled, and stems cut

- 6 radishes, cleaned, peeled, and quartered
- 3 tbsp. melted butter
- 2 tsp. toasted sesame oil
- 2 tbsp. raw honey
- 1\4 cup rice vinegar
- 2 tbsp. white miso paste
- 1\4 cup onions, finely chopped
- 1 tbsp. water
- 1 large apple. peeled, cored, and sliced into thin sticks

DIRECTIONS:

1. In a bowl, whisk together the 1 tablespoon sugar, 1 tablespoon mirin, 1 tablespoon rice vinegar, 1\4 cup white miso paste, and the 1 chopped spring onion. Place the chicken in an airtight container and coat evenly with the marinade. Seal the container and chill in the fridge for 12-24 hours before using.

2. Set the oven to preheat at 450°F.

3. Combine the salt, pepper, 2 spring onions, 3 tablespoons of oil, sprouts, and radishes in a bowl, toss until evenly coated.

4. Remove the chicken from the fridge, use a basting brush to brush off most of the marinade before arranging the chicken, skin side up, on a lightly oiled baking sheet. Clean your basting brush and use the melted butter to coat the chicken skin. Place the vegetables on the other half of the sheet and bake in the oven for 20 minutes before turning the vegetables with a spatula and turning the pan. Bake for an additional 5-10 minutes or until the chicken is properly cooked and crispy.

5. While the chicken is cooking, prepare your chicken sauce. In a large bowl, whisk together the sesame oil, honey, rice vinegar, miso paste, chopped onion, and water.

6. Remove the chicken and vegetables from the oven, and drizzle with the sauce before serving. Top with the fresh apple slices if desired.

BUTTERY VINAIGRETTE CHICKEN

COOK TIME: 50 MINS | MAKES: 4 SERVINGS

INGREDIENTS:

- 1\2 cup melted butter
- 2 tsp. worcestershire sauce
- 1 cup balsamic vinegar
- 1 tsp. liquid smoke
- 1\2 tsp. chili sauce
- 1 tbsp. salt
- 2 tbsp. brown sugar

- 1\2 lemon, squeezed
- 1 tsp. freshly ground black pepper
- 2 sprigs of fresh rosemary, finely chopped
- 4 chicken breasts
- olive oil
- extra rosemary
- 1 lemon, quartered

DIRECTIONS:

1. In a large bowl, combine the melted butter, Worcestershire sauce, vinegar, liquid smoke, chili sauce, salt, sugar, lemon juice, pepper, and rosemary. Whisk until everything is properly mixed. Add the chicken breasts and toss until the chicken is evenly coated.

2. Pour the chicken with all the marinade into an airtight container and chill for at least 4 hours, or overnight before using.

3. Set the oven to preheat at 350°F. Lightly coat a baking sheet with olive oil.

4. Remove the chicken from the marinade and set the extra marinade aside for basting. Arrange the chicken on the prepared sheet, skin side up, and bake for 50 minutes, basting at regular intervals throughout until the chicken is properly cooked and the skin is nice and crispy.

5. Plate and serve with an extra sprig of rosemary and fresh lemon on the side.

CORIANDER CHICKEN WITH CURRIED CARROTS

COOK TIME: 50 MINS | MAKES: 6 SERVINGS

INGREDIENTS:

Spice mixture:
- 1\2 tsp. salt
- 1\2 tsp. smoked paprika
- 1 tsp. ground cumin
- 1 tsp. ground oreganum
- 2 tbsp. shredded fresh ginger
- 1 green chili, diced
- 2 tsp. crushed garlic
- 3 tbsp. apple cider vinegar
- 3\4 cup lime juice
- 1\3 cup soy sauce
- 1\2 cup olive oil
- 1\4 cup fresh estragon leaves

- 1 cup fresh mint leaves
- 1 cup coriander leaves
- 3 lb. chicken cuts of choice

Curried carrots mixture:
- 1\2 tsp. black pepper
- 1\2 tsp. salt
- 1\2 tsp. smoked paprika
- 1\2 tsp. ground cumin
- 2 tsp. turmeric powder
- 2 tbsp. olive oil
- 11\2 pounds baby carrots
- 3\4 cup tangy mayonnaise

DIRECTIONS:

1. In a blender, combine all the ingredients for the spice mixture and pulse to form a paste. Reserve 3\4 cups of the paste for later. In a large bowl, toss the chicken and remaining paste until evenly coated. Transfer to an airtight container and chill for at least 5 hours or overnight before using.

2. Prepare a baking sheet by lining it with tin foil and place a rack over the sheet. Set the oven to preheat at 375°F.

3. In a large bowl, combine the pepper, salt, smoked paprika, cumin, turmeric, olive oil, and baby carrots. Mix until everything is properly combined and the carrots are evenly coated.

4. Arrange the marinated chicken on the rack and place the coated baby carrots on the tinfoil underneath, spreading them out. Place in the oven and bake for 30 minutes. After 30 minutes, stir the carrots and turn up the heat to 450°F. Bake for an additional 15-20 minutes or until the chicken is properly cooked and the baby carrots are fork-tender.

5. Beat the set aside paste with the mayonnaise and serve as a sauce over the chicken.

CILANTRO-CRUSTED CHICKEN & CHICKPEAS

COOK TIME: 40 MINS | MAKES: 3-4 SERVINGS

INGREDIENTS:

- 1 tsp. cumin seeds
- 1 tsp. cilantro seeds
- 1 tsp. peppercorns
- 1 tbsp. sesame seeds
- 1\2 lb. chicken cuts of choice
- olive oil
- 6 tbsp. melted butter
- 2 tsp. salt

- 1 tsp. dried rosemary
- 4 cups cleaned and cut cauliflower
- 1 cup chickpeas, rinsed and drained
- black pepper
- 1\2 lemon, juiced
- 1\4 cup chopped mint leaves
- 1\2 cup pomegranate seeds

DIRECTIONS:

1. Set the oven to preheat at 450°F.

2. In a hot wok with no oil, roast the cumin, cilantro, and peppercorns until their flavor is released. You will be able to smell when they are ready. Tossing all the time to prevent burning. Place the roasted spices in a blender and pulse once, leaving the mixture coarse. Pour the spice mixture into a small bowl and mix with the sesame seeds.

3. In a small bowl, whisk together 1 tsp. olive oil, melted butter, salt, and dried rosemary. With clean hands, massage the butter mixture into the chicken. Giving it an even coat. Sprinkle the spice mixture over a plate and press the chicken into the spice, giving it a nice coarse coating.

4. In a large bowl, combine the cauliflower, chickpeas, 2 tablespoons olive oil, and season with salt and pepper to taste. Toss until evenly coated.

5. Lightly coat a baking sheet with olive oil. Arrange the coated chicken on one half of the pan and scatter the chickpeas and cauliflower on the other half. Place the sheet in the oven and bake for 20 minutes before turning the cauliflower and chickpeas with a spatula and baking for an additional 20 minutes, or until the chicken is properly cooked. The chickpeas should be crispy and the cauliflower fork-tender.

6. In a small glass bowl, whisk together the lemon juice, mint leaves, and pomegranate seeds. Sprinkle over the chicken before serving.

MEXICAN LIME CHICKEN

COOK TIME: 60 MINS | MAKES: 6-8 SERVINGS

INGREDIENTS:

- freshly ground black pepper
- himalayan salt
- 1\3 cup fresh lime juice
- 3\4 cup olive oil
- 1\2 cup fresh oreganum leaves
- 4 garlic cloves, peeled
- 1 whole chicken (3-4 lb.)
- 2 shallots, peeled and quartered
- 2 lb. carrots, peeled and cut into strips

- 2 lb. baby potatoes, peeled and halved
- 2 1\2 cups chicken stock

DIRECTIONS:

1. In a blender, pulse 3\4 teaspoon black pepper, 1\2 teaspoon Salt, 1\3 cup lime juice, 1\2 cup olive oil, 1\2 cup oreganum leaves, and the 4 garlic cloves until just blended into a paste. Do not over mix.

2. In a large bowl, massage the chicken with the spice paste to coat in an even layer. Use plastic wrap to cover the bowl. Chill for at least 2 hours or up to 25 hours before use.

3. Set the oven to preheat at 450°F.

4. In a large bowl, combine the shallots, carrots, baby potatoes, 1\2 teaspoon salt, 1\2 teaspoon pepper, and the rest of the olive oil, 1\4 cup. Mix until evenly coated.

5. Lightly coat a baking sheet with olive and place the marinated chicken in the middle. Arrange the coated vegetables around the chicken. You can use a separate sheet for the vegetables if there isn't enough space.

6. Place the sheet or sheets in the oven and bake for 15 minutes. Lower the heat to 375°F and remove the chicken and vegetables from the oven. Pour the chicken stock over the chicken into the pan. If you are using two pans, divide the stock between the sheets.

7. Return the chicken and vegetables to the oven and bake for an additional 45 minutes or until the chicken is properly cooked and the vegetables are nice and crispy.

CHICKEN-SAUSAGE APPLE BAKE

COOK TIME: 40 MINUTES | MAKES: 4 SERVINGS

INGREDIENTS:

- 3\4 tsp. black pepper
- 1 tsp. himalayan salt
- 1\4 cup balsamic vinegar
- 6 tbsp. olive oil
- 2 tsp. crushed rosemary
- 2 small fennel bulbs, diced. keep the sprigs for later.
- 2 sweet apples, cored sliced
- 1 lb. sausage links
- 2 pouches, ready-made rice

DIRECTIONS:

1. Set the oven to preheat at 375°F.

2. In a bowl, combine the pepper, salt, vinegar, olive oil, and rosemary.

3. In a separate bowl, mix the sliced fennel bulbs, apples, sausages, and 6 tablespoons of the spice mixture. Set the rest aside.

4. Lightly coat a baking sheet with olive oil. Heap the rice in the middle of the sheet and place the apple and sausage mixture on top. Pour the rest of the spice mixture over everything. Place in the oven and bake for 40 minutes or until the sausages are properly cooked and the apples are a crispy brown.

5. Divide and plate the cooked food. Sprinkle with the chopped fennel sprigs and serve.

FIERY GLAZED DRUMSTICKS

COOK TIME: 40 MINS | MAKES: 4 SERVINGS

INGREDIENTS:

- 1\2 tsp. salt
- 2 tbsp. raw honey
- 1\4 tsp. ground allspice
- 5 sprigs fresh thyme
- 3 green red chilies
- 2 cloves garlic
- 3 spring onions, chopped
- 5 tsp. grated fresh ginger
- 3 tbsp. packed brown sugar
- 3 tbsp. lime juice
- 1\4 cup soy sauce
- 1\4 cup olive oil
- 1 tsp. chili flakes
- 1\3 tsp. cayenne pepper
- 12 chicken drumsticks
- 1 lime sliced into wedges
- 1 green chili, chopped

DIRECTIONS:

1. In a blender, pulse the salt, honey, allspice, thyme, chopped chilies, garlic, spring onions, ginger, sugar, lime juice, soy sauce, olive oil, chili flakes, and cayenne pepper to form a smooth paste. Place the drumsticks in an airtight container and coat with the spice paste. Chill for at least 4 hours or overnight before use.

2. Line a baking sheet with tinfoil and place a wire rack over the sheet. Set the oven to preheat at 425°F.

3. Remove the chicken from the marinade and use a basting brush to remove the majority of the sauce. Arrange the drumsticks on the wire rack above the sheet. They should not be touching. Place the sheet in the oven and bake for 30-40 minutes. Turning the drumsticks halfway through. Bake until the chicken is properly cooked.

4. Plate the drumsticks and garnish with the chopped chili. Serve with lime wedges on the side.

ASIAN FIVE-SPICE CHICKEN

COOK TIME: 35 MINS | MAKES: 4-6 SERVINGS

INGREDIENTS:

- 1 fennel bulb with sprigs
- 3\4 lb. yams
- 1 purple onion
- 2 large granny smith apples
- 1 1\2 tsp. himalayan salt.
- 1\2 tsp. black pepper
- 2 tbsp. olive oil
- 6 chicken thighs
- 1 tbsp. honey

- 1 tbsp. english mustard
- 2 tbsp. salted butter, melted
- 1 1\2 tsp. chinese five-spice
- fennel leaves, chopped

DIRECTIONS:

1. Set the oven to preheat at 425°F.

2. Clean, peel, and trim the fennel bulb before cutting it into 1\4-inch wedges. Set aside the fennel sprigs for later. Clean, peel and slice the yams into 1\4-inch slices. Peel and slice the onion into 1\4-inch wedges. Peel, core, and cut the apple into 1\4-inch wedges. Toss them all into a large bowl and coat with the salt, pepper, and olive oil.

3. Grease a baking sheet with a light layer of olive oil and spread the vegetables over the sheet. Arrange the chicken on top of the vegetables.

4. In a small bowl, whisk together the honey, mustard, melted butter, and five-spice. Use a basting brush to evenly coat all the chicken with the five-spice mixture.

5. Place the baking sheet in the oven and bake for 15 minutes. Remove the pan from the oven and use the sauce on the sheet to baste the chicken and vegetables. Return the sheet to the oven and bake for another 15-20 minutes until the chicken is properly cooked and the skin is nice and crispy.

6. Remove the sheet from the oven and baste once more before garnishing with the fennel leaves and serving.

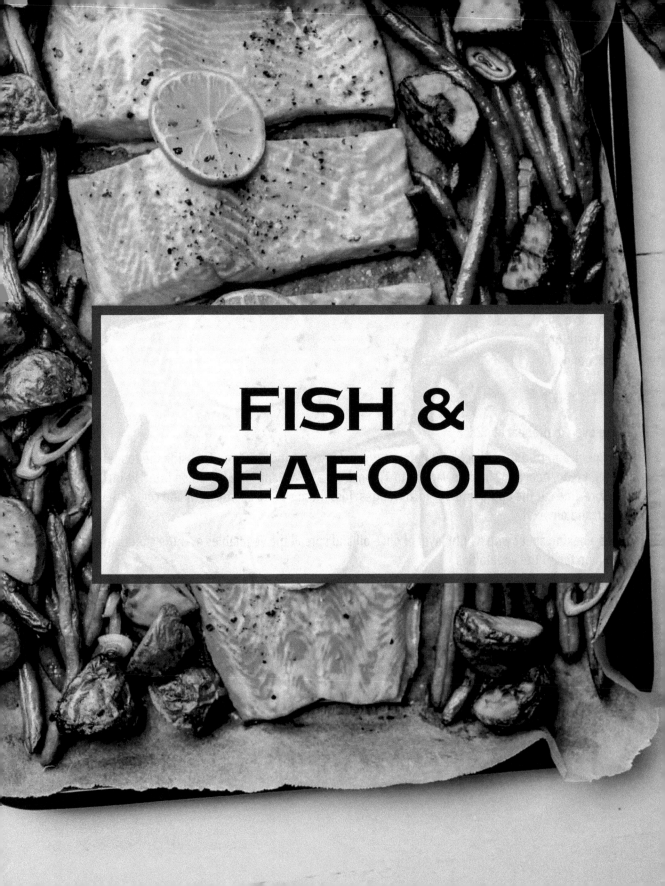

FISH & SEAFOOD

RICH SEAFOOD TOSS UP

COOK TIME: 35 MINS | MAKES: 4 SERVINGS

INGREDIENTS:

- 2 lemons, halved
- 2 shallots, cut into 1-inch wedges
- 12 oz. baby potatoes
- 3 tbsp. olive oil.
- 1 1\2 tsp. cajun seafood boil seasoning
- 2 lb. littleneck clams, scrubbed
- 12 oz. smoked pork sausage, sliced (2-inch rounds)
- 1 lb. fresh mussels in shells, scrubbed

- 1\2 cup dry white wine
- 2 tbsp. chopped parsley
- 1 1\2 tsp. worcestershire sauce
- 1 tbsp. hot sauce
- 1\4 cup salted butter, melted
- 2 tsp. crushed garlic
- lemon wedges

DIRECTIONS:

1. Place two racks in the oven on the second slot from the bottom and the second slot from the top. Set the oven to preheat at 450°F. Line 2 baking sheets with tin foil.

2. In a large bowl, combine the lemons, shallots, baby potatoes, olive oil, 1 1\2 teaspoons seafood boil seasoning. Mix until evenly coated. Spread the seasoned vegetables out on the prepared baking sheet and bake at the bottom of the oven for 25 minutes, or until a knife can be easily inserted into the potatoes.

3. Place the clams on the second baking sheet and bake at the top of the oven for 7-9 minutes or until the clams just start to open.

4. Remove both sheets from the oven when they are done. Turn the potatoes and sprinkle the sausage rounds on top. Arrange the mussels over the clams and pour the wine over the mussels and clams. Return both sheets to the oven and bake for an additional 8 minutes, or until the mussels have opened. Remove and throw away any mussels and clams that have not opened.

5. In a glass bowl, whisk together the parsley, Worcestershire sauce, hot sauce, melted butter, and crushed garlic. Take the baked potato and sausage mixture and spread it in an even layer over the mussels and clams. Pour the butter mixture over everything and serve with lemon wedges on the side.

SPICY ROASTED SHRIMP COCKTAIL

COOK TIME: 25 MINS | MAKES: 4 SERVINGS

INGREDIENTS:

- 3 poblano peppers, seeded and sliced
- 1 red onion, peeled and sliced
- 1 tbsp. olive oil
- 2 tsp. chili flakes
- 1\2 tsp. salt
- 1\2 tsp. black pepper
- 1 tsp. garlic powder
- 1 lb. shrimp, shelled and deveined
- 4 radishes, sliced
- 1\2 tsp. salt
- 1\2 tsp. pepper
- 3 tbsp. lime juice
- 5 oz. mixed salad greens
- 1 avocado, thinly sliced

DIRECTIONS:

1. Set the oven to preheat at 450°F. Lightly coat a baking sheet with olive oil.

2. Combine the chilies, sliced onion, olive oil, chili flakes, salt, pepper, and garlic powder in a bowl. Mix until evenly coated before spreading it out on the prepared baking sheet. Bake in the oven for 20 minutes.

3. Arrange the shrimp between the onion mixture and return the sheet to the oven. Bake for an additional 5 minutes or until the shrimp blush (turn a light shade of pink) and form a C. Set the sheet on the counter and allow the shrimp to rest for 5 minutes.

4. Toss together the cooled shrimp mixture, radishes, salt, pepper, lime juice, and salad greens in a large bowl, until evenly coated.

5. Use 4 large cocktail glasses and scoop even amounts of the shrimp salad into each. Garnish with the avocado slices and serve.

SOUR CREAM SHRIMP TORTILLAS

COOK TIME: 10 MINS | MAKES: 4 SERVINGS

INGREDIENTS:

- 1\4 tsp. table salt
- 2 tbsp. lemon juice
- 3 cups shredded savoy cabbage
- 1 1\2 lb. medium shrimp deveined, and deshelled
- 1\4 tsp. himalayan salt
- 1 tbsp. chili powder
- 1 lemon, sliced into wedges
- 1 jalapeno, sliced
- 4 spring onions, chopped and divided between green and white

- 1 1\2 cups frozen corn kernels
- 2 tbsp. olive oil
- 2 avocados
- 1\2 cup sour cream
- 1\4 tsp. black pepper
- 1\4 tsp. himalayan salt
- 1\2 cup coriander leaves
- 8 soft corn tortillas, heated

DIRECTIONS:

1. Set the oven to preheat at 425°F with the wire rack in the middle of the oven.

2. In a large bowl, toss the salt and lemon juice with the cabbage and set aside while you prepare the rest of the dish. It will marinate while you work.

3. Coat the shrimp with the Himalayan salt and chili powder before placing them on a lightly oiled baking sheet. Arrange the lemon wedges, Jalapeno, the white parts of the spring onions, and the frozen corn around the shrimp. Sprinkle everything with 2 tablespoons of olive oil. Place the sheet in the oven and bake for 10 minutes or until the shrimp blush, (turn a light shade of pink.) Cooked shrimp will form a C.

4. In a food processor, pulse the avocados, sour cream, salt, and pepper to form a lump-free paste. Transfer half of the paste to the marinated cabbage and mix with a wooden spoon until properly combined and coated. Use the remaining avocado mixture as a spread on the inside of the tortillas before dividing the contents of the sheet pan evenly amongst the tortillas, leaving the lemon wedges on the sheet. Place the cabbage mixture on top of the shrimp and garnish evenly with the green part of the spring onions. Squeeze the lemon wedges over the tortillas, fold and serve.

(Quick Tip) You can place a second rack in the bottom of the oven to heat the tortillas while the shrimp cook.

BUTTERY CRUMBED MUSSELS

COOK TIME: 12 MINS | MAKES: 4 SERVINGS

INGREDIENTS:

- 1 large purple onion, sliced
- 2 fennel bulbs, trimmed and cut with the sprigs set aside
- 3 tomatoes, each sliced into 6 wedges
- 2 tbsp. Olive oil
- 1\2 tsp. Salt
- 1\2 tsp. Black pepper

- 2 lb. mussels, scrubbed
- 6 tbsp. Butter, cubed
- 1 cup seasoned bread crumbs
- 1 lemon for sprinkling

DIRECTIONS:

1. Set the oven to preheat at 450°F and lightly grease a baking sheet with olive oil.

2. In a large bowl, toss together the onion, fennel bulbs, tomatoes, olive oil, salt, and pepper.

3. Place the mussels on the prepared baking sheet and sprinkle with 4 tablespoons of the cubed butter. Arrange the coated vegetables around the mussels, including the reserved fennel sprigs.

4. In a medium bowl, combine the remaining butter with the bread crumbs and use your fingers to work the butter through. Sprinkle the breadcrumbs over everything on the baking sheet and bake in the oven for 10-12 minutes or until the mussels open. Throw away any mussels that have not opened, as unopened means inedible. Serve the opened mussels and vegetables with a sprinkling of lemon juice.

LEMON-GARLIC SHRIMP & COURGETTE FRIES

COOK TIME: 12 MINS | MAKES: 4 SERVINGS

INGREDIENTS:

- 1\2 tsp. salt
- 1 clove garlic, peeled
- 1 large egg
- 1 large egg yolk
- 1 cup melted butter
- 1 lemon, zest, and juice
- 1\2 tsp. salt
- 1\2 tsp. pepper
- 1 1\2 tbsp. french mustard
- 1 1\2 tbsp. lemon juice

- 3 tsp. crushed garlic
- 3 tbsp. olive oil
- 1 1\4 lb. shrimp, deshelled and deveined
- 1\2 cup all-purpose flour
- 1 tbsp. water
- 2 large eggs
- 1\4 cup parmesan cheese
- 1 cup seasoned bread crumbs
- 1 lb. courgettes, peeled and cut into fries
- chopped parsley for garnish

DIRECTIONS:

1. Set the oven to preheat at 425°F. Lightly spray a baking sheet with baking spray before lining the pan with tin foil and coating the tinfoil with another light layer of spray.

2. In a blender, mince the salt and garlic glove. Add the egg, and egg yolk till properly combined. While the mixture is blending, gradually drizzle in the melted butter to form your sauce. Transfer the mixture to a separate bowl and whisk in the lemon juice and zest. Cover the bowl with cling wrap and allow it to rest on the counter while you prepare the rest of the dish.

3. In a large bowl, whisk together the salt, pepper, mustard, lemon juice, garlic, and olive oil. Mix in the shrimp and set aside on the counter.

4. You will need 3 bowls to prepare the courgette fries. Place the flour in the first bowl. In the second bowl, beat the water and eggs. In the third bowl, combine the bread crumbs and parmesan. Take your cut courgette fries and roll them in the flour. Dip them in the egg mixture before coating them generously in the bread crumbs.

5. Place your prepared Courgettes on half of the prepared baking sheet and arrange the shrimp on the other half. Place the sheet in the oven and bake for 10-12 minutes until the shrimp curl into a C and the courgette fries are nice and crispy. Remove from the oven and plate before pouring the garlic sauce over the shrimp and garnishing with parsley.

(Quick Tip) Preheating the oven at the start is crucial to cook time in this recipe.

SPICY TILAPIA WRAPS

COOK TIME: 10 MINS | MAKES: 4 SERVINGS

INGREDIENTS:

- 1 tsp. crushed garlic
- 1\4 tsp. salt
- 1 1\2 tsp. fresh lime juice
- 1 tsp. lime zest
- 3 tbsp. sour cream
- 3 tbsp. tangy mayonnaise
- 1\4 cup coriander leaves, chopped
- 1\2 cup spring onions, sliced
- 1\4 tsp. garlic powder
- 1\4 tsp. cayenne pepper

- 1\2 tsp. smoked paprika
- 1 tsp. cumin
- 1 tsp. ground coriander seeds
- 1 1\2 lb. tilapia fillets
- 8 corn tortilla wraps
- 2 cups pre-made coleslaw
- 1\2 cup sliced shallots
- 1 cup tomatoes, sliced
- 2 limes, quartered

DIRECTIONS:

1. Set the oven to preheat at 425°F. Line a baking sheet with a light layer of baking spray.

2. Whisk together the garlic, salt, lime juice, zest, sour cream, mayonnaise, coriander leaves, and spring onions. Store in the fridge while you prepare the rest of the food.

3. In a small bowl, whisk together the garlic powder, cayenne pepper, smoked paprika, cumin, and ground coriander seeds to form the spice mixture.

4. Place the filets on a wooden board and sprinkle both sides with your prepared spice mixture before placing the fish on the prepared sheet and baking for 10 minutes or until the fish can easily break apart. Remove the pan from the oven and allow to cool for a few minutes on the counter while you warm the wraps in the oven.

5. In a large bowl, break the fish up with a fork.

6. Spread the sour cream mixture over the cooked wraps and divide the fish evenly between the wraps.

7. Top with the coleslaw, and chopped vegetables. Sprinkle with juice from the lime wedges before folding and serving.

ASIAN BAKED SALMON

COOK TIME: 27 MINS| MAKES: 4 SERVINGS

INGREDIENTS:

- 1\2 tsp. salt
- 1 tbsp. olive oil
- 4 oz. green chilies, chopped
- 1 bunch spring onions, sliced
- 5 celery stalks, chopped
- 4 salmon filets, skinned
- 2 tbsp. soy sauce
- 1\4 cup peanuts
- steamed pok choi

DIRECTIONS:

1. Set the oven to preheat at 450°F and lightly coat two baking sheets with baking spray.

2. In a large bowl, toss together the salt, olive oil, chilies, spring onions, and celery. Fan the seasoned vegetables out on a prepared baking sheet and place in the oven for 15 minutes, stirring when half the time is up.

3. Coat the salmon fillets with soy sauce before placing them on the second baking sheet. Bake the salmon in the oven with the vegetables for an additional 12 minutes or until the fish begins to darken. You can stir the vegetables again if they start to burn.

4. Garnish the salmon and vegetables with peanuts and serve on a bed of steamed pok choi.

SPICY SPANISH SEAFOOD RICE

COOK TIME: 22 MINS | MAKES: 4 SERVINGS

INGREDIENTS:

- 1 cup arborio rice
- 1\2 tsp. salt
- 1\2 tsp. pepper
- 1 small onion, chopped
- 2 tsp. crushed garlic
- 3\4 tsp. smoked paprika
- 1\4 tsp. cayenne pepper
- 1 bay leaf, torn in half
- 1 tsp. fried saffron, crushed

- 2 1\2 cups chicken broth
- 6 oz. spicy sausage, cut into 1\4-inch rounds
- 2 sweet chili peppers, roasted and chopped with the seeds removed
- 1 cup canned tomatoes, drained and chopped
- 12 shrimp, peeled, and deveined
- 2 tbsp. olive oil
- 12 clams, scrubbed
- chopped parsley for garnish

DIRECTIONS:

1. Set the oven to preheat at 350°F and lightly spray a rimmed baking sheet with baking spray.

2. Fan the rice out on the prepared baking sheet and roast in the preheated oven for 5 minutes.

3. In a large bowl, whisk together the salt, pepper, chopped onion, garlic, smoked paprika, cayenne pepper, bay leaf halves, saffron, and chicken broth.

4. Pour the spice broth over the roasted rice on the baking sheet. You can use a wooden spoon or whisk to mix it through. Seal the sheet with tin foil and carefully return it to the oven for 15 minutes. When the 15 minutes are up, remove the pan from the oven and leave it uncovered on the counter while you prepare the rest of the dish.

5. Place the sausage rounds, chilies, and tomatoes onto the rice mixture and stir through. Season with a pinch of salt and pepper. Coat the shrimp with olive oil before arranging them with the clams on top of the rice.

6. Place the sheet in the oven and bake for 12 minutes or until the shrimp curl into a C and the clams open. Pick out and throw away any clams that have not opened. Garnish the whole dish with parsley and serve.

BUTTERY SPINACH & LEMON SCALLOPS

COOK TIME: 42 MINS | MAKES: 4 SERVINGS

INGREDIENTS:

- 5 tbsp. olive oil
- 2 lemons, sliced (1\4-inch slices)
- black pepper
- himalayan salt
- 2 bunches of spinach, cleaned and trimmed
- 1 1\4 lb. scallops, side muscle removed
- 1 tbsp. melted butter
- chopped parsley for garnish
- 1 lemon, squeezed

DIRECTIONS:

1. Line a baking sheet with greaseproof paper and set the oven to preheat at 325°F.

2. Use 1 tablespoon of olive oil to coat the lemon slices. Season them with a pinch of salt and pepper before placing them separately on the prepared baking sheet and baking for 20 minutes before turning and baking for another 10 minutes. The edges should just be starting to scorch. Remove the baked lemon slices from the sheet and leave to cool.

3. Set the oven to 400°F.

4. Coat the cleaned spinach with 2 tablespoons of olive oil. Season with a pinch of salt and pepper. In a separate bowl, coat the scallops with 2 tablespoons of olive oil.

5. Arrange the scallops on the sheet with greaseproof paper and brush the tops with the melted butter. Place the sheet in the oven and bake for 7 minutes. Remove the pan from the oven and push the scallops to the side, making room for the spinach and lemon slices on the other half of the sheet. Return the baking sheet to the oven for an additional 5 minutes or until the scallops are brown and the spinach has reduced in size.

6. Plate and garnish with the parsley before sprinkling with the extra lemon juice.

SWEET & SOUR CASHEW SALMON

COOK TIME: 15 MINS| MAKES: 4 SERVINGS

INGREDIENTS:

- 2 tbsp. canola oil
- 1 tbsp. chopped fresh ginger
- 2 garlic cloves, chopped
- 1 onion, chopped
- 2 tbsp. maple syrup
- 1\4 cup chopped roasted cashews
- zest from 1 lime
- 1\2 tsp. chili paste

- salt pepper
- 1 tbsp. maple syrup
- 1 tbsp. miso sauce
- 1 1\2 lb. salmon fillet, skin removed
- 1 tbsp. canola oil
- 3\4 lb. sugar snap peas
- cooked basmati rice for serving

DIRECTIONS:

1. Set the oven to preheat at 425°F and place a wire rack in the middle of the oven. Line a baking sheet with greaseproof paper.

2. With the stove plate on high, heat the canola oil and add the ginger, garlic and chopped onion. Stir until everything is nicely browned. Stir in the syrup and cashews, allowing the mixture to simmer for a minute or two before transferring to a bowl. Add the zest and chili paste, mixing through. Season with a pinch of salt and pepper, set aside.

3. In a small glass bowl, whisk together the maple syrup and miso sauce. Place the salmon filets on the prepared baking sheet and use a basting brush to coat them with the miso syrup. Place the sheet in the oven for 4 minutes.

4. Coat the snap peas with oil before arranging them around the salmon and baking for an additional 4 minutes until the fish is properly cooked. Top with the lime sauce and serve on a bed of basmati rice.

WINE & HERB BAKED SNAPPER

COOK TIME: 35 MINS | MAKES: 4-6 SERVINGS

INGREDIENTS:

- 1 (4 lb.) snapper
- 3 tbsp. melted butter
- salt
- pepper
- 2 lemons, sliced
- 1 fennel bulb, trimmed and sliced
- 2 rosemary sprigs
- 1 1\2 cups dry white wine
- 2 tbsp. red wine vinegar
- 1\2 cup coriander leaves, chopped
- 1 cup parsley chopped

- 1\4 tsp. pepper flakes
- 1 1\2 tsp. ground cumin
- 1 tsp crushed garlic
- 6 tbsp. olive oil

DIRECTIONS:

1. Line a baking sheet with tin foil that's about 4-inches bigger than the sheet on all sides. Set the oven to preheat at 400°F.

2. Prepare your fish by making 4 long cuts on both sides of the snapper. Use a basting brush to evenly coat the fish with the melted butter and season with a pinch of salt and pepper.

3. Layer the lemon and fennel slices inside the fish with the sprigs of rosemary. Use all of the lemon and fennel slices that do not fit inside the fish to create a layer on the tin foil and place the fish on top. Fold the foil to create a container and pour the wine over the fish. Place the sheet in the oven and bake for 30-35 minutes until the fish is nicely browned.

4. In a blender, pulse the red wine vinegar, coriander leaves, parsley, pepper flakes, cumin, and crushed garlic until chunky. Do not over pulse at this stage. Drizzle in the olive oil and pulse to form a sauce. Season to taste with salt and pepper.

5. Remove the fish from the oven and throw away the fennel and lemon slices. Serve with the sauce on the side.

CRUMBED TILAPIA FILETS

COOK TIME: 12 MINS | MAKES: 4 SERVINGS

INGREDIENTS:

- 4 tilapia filets
- 1\4 tsp. black pepper
- 3\8 tsp. himalayan salt
- 1\3 cup corn flour
- 1 large egg
- 1 tbsp. water
- 1 cup seasoned bread crumbs
- 2 tbsp. olive oil

- 1 lb. asparagus, trimmed
- 1 tbsp. spring onions, chopped
- 1 tbsp. dill pickle relish
- 1\4 cup tangy mayonnaise

DIRECTIONS:

1. Place a baking sheet in the oven and leave it there while the oven is set to preheat at 450°F.

2. Season the tilapia with 1\2 teaspoons each of pepper and salt.

3. Place the corn flour in a large bowl. In a separate bowl, whisk together the water and egg. Spread the bread crumbs out over a plate. Coat the filets in the corn flour before drenching them in the egg mixture and giving them an even coat with the bread crumbs.

4. Using oven gloves, carefully remove the heated pan from the oven. Coat with baking spray and sprinkle with olive oil. Moving the pan to coat it evenly. Arrange both the coated fish and trimmed asparagus on the baking sheet and sprinkle the remaining salt over the asparagus. Return the sheet to the oven and bake for 12 minutes, turning everything halfway through, or until the fish is properly cooked and the asparagus is fork-tender.

5. Whisk together the spring onions, pickle relish, and mayonnaise to serve on the side of the fish and asparagus as a dipping sauce.

FULL BAKED SALMON LUNCH

COOK TIME: 35 MINS | MAKES: 4 SERVINGS

INGREDIENTS:

- 3\4 tsp. himalayan salt
- 3\4 tsp. black pepper
- 2 tbsp. olive oil
- 1 lb. fingerling potatoes halved
- 1 lb. haricot verts, trimmed
- 4 salmon filets, skin removed
- 1 lemon, halved
- 3 sprigs of fresh rosemary for garnish

DIRECTIONS:

1. Set the oven to preheat at 425°F and line a large baking sheet with tin foil.

2. In a large bowl, use 1\4 teaspoon each of the salt and pepper, and half of the olive oil to evenly coat the potatoes. Arrange the coated potatoes, face down, on the baking sheet, and bake in the oven for 20-25 minutes or until a knife can slide in and out with ease.

3. In the bowl you used to coat the potatoes, combine the haricot verts with the remaining olive oil and 1\4 tsp each of the salt and pepper. Mix to give an even coat.

4. Remove the potatoes from the oven when they are tender and set the oven to broil.

5. Use the remaining salt and pepper to season the salmon. Push the potatoes to the sides and arrange the seasoned salmon in the middle of the baking sheet. Arrange the haricot verts amongst the potatoes. Squeeze half the lemon over everything on the pan.

6. Take the other half of the lemon and cut it into thin slices to arrange on top of the fish. Lastly, garnish the Salmon with the rosemary sprigs and broil in the oven for 10 minutes or until the Salmon is properly cooked and the vegetables are nice and crisp.

MEDITERRANEAN BAKED BASS FILETS

COOK TIME: 15 MINS | MAKES: 4 SERVINGS

INGREDIENTS:

- 1\3 cup green olives, pips removed
- 1\2 lb. baby tomatoes, quartered
- 4 oz. haricot verts, trimmed
- 1 cup canned chickpeas, drained
- 1 cup fresh corn kernels
- 1 tsp. salt
- 1 tsp. pepper
- 2 tbsp. olive oil

- 4 bass filets, skin removed
- 4 sprigs of fresh oreganum

DIRECTIONS:

1. Set the oven to preheat at 425°F and measure either a piece of greaseproof paper or tin foil that is about 4-inches longer than the baking sheet on all sides.

2. In a large bowl, toss together the olives, tomatoes, haricot verts, chickpeas, corn kernels, 1\2 teaspoon salt, 1\2 teaspoon pepper, and olive oil until evenly coated. On a chopping board, season the filets with the remaining salt and pepper.

3. Spread the seasoned vegetables over the prepared tin foil\greaseproof paper on the baking sheet to create a bed for the filets, nestle the fish in the bed, and garnish with the oreganum sprigs. Fold the foil\greaseproof paper over to seal the dish. This will prevent the fish from drying out.

4. Place the sheet with the sealed fish in the oven and bake for 12-15 minutes or until the fish is browned.

HONEY & MUSTARD GLAZED SALMON FILETS

COOK TIME: 26 MINS | MAKES: 8 SERVINGS

INGREDIENTS:

- 1\4 cup french mustard
- 1 tsp. white wine vinegar
- 2 tbsp. raw honey
- 10 sprigs of fresh thyme
- 8 salmon filets with the skin still on
- 1\2 tsp. black pepper
- 1 tsp. salt
- 2 tsp. crushed thyme
- 1 lemon, thinly sliced

DIRECTIONS:

1. Set the oven to preheat at 450°F with the wire rack in the middle of the oven, and line a baking sheet with greaseproof paper.

2. In a small glass bowl, whisk together the mustard, honey, and wine vinegar. Dip the filets in the glaze to give them an even coat.

3. Place the thyme sprigs in a row on the prepared baking sheet. Arrange the glazed salmon filets over the sprigs and brush the rest of the glaze over the filets. Sprinkle the crushed thyme, pepper, and salt over the glazed fish and garnish with the lemon slices.

4. Place the sheet in the oven and bake for 26 minutes or until the salmon is properly cooked to taste. Serve immediately.

SPANISH-STYLE COD BAKE

COOK TIME: 23 MINS | MAKES: 4 SERVINGS

INGREDIENTS:

- olive oil
- 1 cup mushrooms, sliced
- 1 purple onion, diced
- 4 oz. spicy sausage, sliced into thin rounds
- 1\2 cup green olives, pitted and chopped
- 1 cup baby tomatoes, halved
- 2 tbsp. tomato puree
- himalayan salt
- black pepper

- 1 lb. haricot verts
- 2 tbsp. water
- 4 cod fillets, skin removed
- 1 tsp. smoked paprika

DIRECTIONS:

1. Set the oven to preheat at 450°F and line a baking sheet with greaseproof paper.

2. In a pan over medium heat, heat 1 tablespoon of olive oil and add the mushrooms and onion. Stir for about 5 minutes or until the mushrooms are fork-tender and the onions are lightly browned. Next add the sausage, olives, tomatoes, and tomato puree. Cook for another five minutes and season with a pinch of salt and pepper. Set aside.

3. In a large bowl, coat the haricot verts with 2 tablespoons of water and seal the container with a lid. Microwave on high for 3 minutes. Drain any excess water. Drizzle with 1 tablespoon of olive oil and toss to coat. Season the fillets with paprika and a pinch of salt and pepper.

4. Arrange the fillets on one half of the baking sheet and the haricot verts on the other half. Bake in the oven for 8-10 minutes or until the fish is properly cooked and the haricot verts are fork-tender.

5. Plate the fish and haricot verts, with the relish on top of the cod.

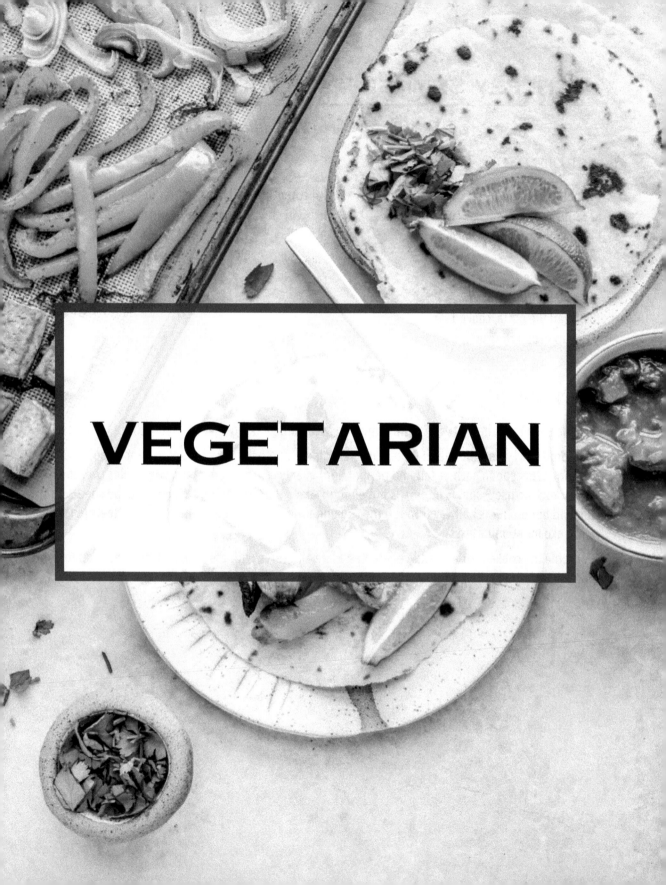

VEGETARIAN

CHEESY SUMMER VEGETABLE FARFALLE

COOK TIME: 20 MINS | MAKES: 4 SERVINGS

INGREDIENTS:

- 1 shallot, chopped
- 2 large summer squash, cubed
- 1 cup baby tomatoes, halved
- olive oil
- himalayan salt
- black pepper
- 8 oz. farfalle pasta, cooked
- 1\2 cup ricotta cheese
- 1\4 cup pecorino cheese, shredded
- 1 cup fresh basil leaves for garnish

DIRECTIONS:

1. Set the oven to preheat at 450°F and lightly grease a large baking sheet with olive oil.

2. In a large bowl, combine the shallots, summer squash, and baby tomatoes with 3 tablespoons of olive oil and 1\2 teaspoon each of salt and pepper until evenly coated. Spread the vegetables over the baking sheet. You can use 2 sheets if there is not enough space. Just remember to alternate the sheets on the top and bottom racks halfway through the cooking time if you do. Place the sheet or sheets in the oven and bake for 20 minutes.

3. Combine the cooked Farfalle and vegetables. Plate and serve with the two kinds of cheese on top and garnish with the basil.

CURRY STUFFED BRINGLES

COOK TIME: 24 MINS | MAKES: 4 SERVINGS

INGREDIENTS:

- olive oil
- 1\2 cup sultanas
- 3 garlic cloves, crushed
- 1\2 tsp. turmeric powder
- 1\2 tsp. curry powder
- salt
- 2 cups water

- 1 cup quick-cooking bulgur
- 2 medium bringles
- black pepper
- 1\2 cup cashews
- 1\2 cup chopped mint for decorating

DIRECTIONS:

1. In a small pot over medium heat, heat 1 tablespoon of olive. Add the sultanas, garlic, turmeric, curry powder, and 1\2 teaspoon salt, mix through and let simmer for 2 minutes before adding the water and bulgur. Stir until the bulgur is just simmering. Cover the pot and let it cook for 15 minutes until the bulgur is soft.

2. While the bulgur is simmering, line a baking sheet with tin foil and set the oven to broil. Halve the bringles lengthwise and remove the seeds. Place the bringles on the baking sheet, open side up and use a basting brush to coat them with 2 tablespoons of olive oil. Sprinkle with a pinch of salt and pepper.

3. Place the sheet in the oven and broil for 7 minutes or until the bringles are fork-tender. Remove the sheet from the oven and cover the bringles with extra foil.

4. Use a fork to separate the cooked curry bulgur and mix in the cashews.

5. Remove the foil from the bringles and spoon even amounts of the curry bulgur into each bringle. Decorate with the mint and serve.

CRISPY BUTTER BASED VEGETABLE PIZZA

COOK TIME: 14 MINS | MAKES: 2-4 SERVINGS

INGREDIENTS:

- premade pizza dough
- all-purpose flour for dusting
- 3 tbsp. melted butter
- olive oil
- 1 cup mozzarella, grated
- 1\4 cup parmesan
- 1 cup ricotta, grated
- 2 small fingerling potatoes, sliced as thin as possible
- salt
- pepper
- 1\4 cup fresh basil leaves, chopped
- 1\3 cup sun-dried tomatoes

DIRECTIONS:

1. Set the oven to preheat at 450°F. A really hot oven is crucial for this recipe, so do not open the oven straight away. Once the oven has reached 450°F, leave the door closed for 15 minutes before using.

2. Line a baking sheet with greaseproof paper.

3. On a lightly floured surface, use a rolling pin to roll your dough into a rectangle to fit your sheet. The dough should hold its shape, if it's too springy you may want to let the dough rest for a while, but this should not happen with store-bought dough.

4. Fit the rolled-out dough into the prepared sheet and use a basting brush to coat the pizza base with the melted butter. Drizzle 1 tablespoon of olive oil over the melted butter. Sprinkle the mozzarella over the base, leaving a 1-inch border at the edges.

5. In a medium bowl, combine the parmesan, ricotta, and 1 tablespoon of olive oil. Spoon the mixture over the mozzarella in heaps. You do not have to spread it.

6. In a bowl, coat the thin potato slices with 1 tablespoon of olive oil. Place the coated potato slices in an even layer over the cheese. It is important to space them evenly. Season the pizza with a pinch of salt and pepper.

7. Place the sheet in the oven for 14 minutes until the base is a crispy brown and the cheese has melted. Take the sheet out of the oven.

8. Garnish the pizza with the basil leaves, sun dried tomatoes, and drizzle with 1 final tablespoon of olive oil before slicing and serving hot.

CHEESY VEGETARIAN FRIKADELLE

COOK TIME: 20 MINS | MAKES: 65 FRIKADELLE

INGREDIENTS:

- 2 cup shredded courgettes
- 2 cans brown legumes, rinsed and drained
- 2 spring onions, chopped
- 1 cup parmesan
- 1 cup mozzarella
- 1\2 tsp. garlic powder
- 1\4 cup ground chia seeds
- 1\4 cup seasoned bread crumbs
- salt
- pepper
- 2 eggs
- 1\4 cup olive oil

DIRECTIONS:

1. Set the oven to preheat at 400°F with the wire rack in the middle of the oven. Lightly coat a baking sheet with olive oil.

2. Using a clean tea towel, wring as much water out of the grated courgettes as possible before placing them in a blender. Add the legumes and spring onions on a pulse to form a chunky paste.

3. In a large bowl, mix together the parmesan, mozzarella, garlic powder, chia seeds, bread crumbs, and a pinch of salt and pepper. Mix in the legume paste and the eggs with a wooden spoon.

4. Use the olive oil to coat your hands and roll the mixture into 65 balls of roughly the same size. Make sure that each ball has a good layer of oil on them. This will help them crisp.

5. Place the sheet in the oven and bake for 10 minutes before turning them and baking for an additional 10 minutes or until they are properly roasted. They can be served straight away or stored in an airtight container in the fridge for no more than 5 days.

SPICY AUTUMN BUTTERNUT BOWLS

COOK TIME: 60 MINS | MAKES: 4 SERVINGS

INGREDIENTS:

- olive oil
- 1 large butternut squash
- black pepper
- himalayan salt
- 1\2 tsp. oregano
- 1\2 tsp. cumin seeds
- 1 cup raw shelled pumpkin seeds
- 1 jalapeno, sliced
- 2 garlic cloves, halved
- 2 tomatillos, husks removed and halved
- 1 small shallot, cut into wedges
- 1\2 cup coriander leaves, chopped
- 1\2 cup parsley, chopped
- 1\2 cup coconut milk
- 3\4 cups vegetable stock
- cooked rice for serving
- 1 lime, quartered

DIRECTIONS:

1. Set the oven to preheat at 400°F. Lightly spray a baking sheet with baking spray.

2. Peel and cut the butternut into 1-inch squares before placing them in a large bowl and coating them with 2 tablespoons olive oil, 1\4 teaspoon of pepper, and 1 teaspoon of salt. Place the coated butternut onto the prepared baking sheet and bake in the oven for 35-40 minutes or until the butternut is fork-tender. You can stir the butternut a few times if it starts to burn.

3. In a dry wok, over medium heat, roast the oregano, cumin seeds, and half of the pumpkin seeds until their fragrance is released. You will be able to smell when they are done. Place them in a glass bowl for later.

4. In the same wok, heat 1 tablespoon of olive oil and add the jalapeno, garlic cloves, tomatillos, and shallots. Stir for 5 minutes until everything is nicely browned. Transfer to a food processor and add the roasted seeds and pulse for a minute or two before adding half of the coriander leaves, parsley, coconut milk, vegetable stock, 1\2 teaspoon salt, 1\4 teaspoon black pepper. Pulse to form a lump-free sauce.

5. Pour the sauce back into the wok and stir over medium heat for 15-20 minutes or until it starts to thicken.

6. Divide the rice and butternut between the bowls and top with the sauce. Garnish with the extra pumpkin seeds and coriander leaves. Serve with lime wedges on the side.

FRENCH ASPARAGUS TART

COOK TIME: 45 MINS | MAKES: 6 SERVINGS

INGREDIENTS:

- 1\4 tsp. salt
- 1 1\2 cups all-purpose flour, extra for dusting
- 1\2 cup cold butter, cubed
- 1\4 cup ice water
- 1\2 cup greek yogurt, unsweetened
- 3-4 cups uncooked rice
- 1 cup cream

- 8 eggs
- 1\2 tsp. salt
- 1\2 tsp. pepper
- 3\4 lb. asparagus, trimmed and blanched

DIRECTIONS:

1. In a blender, mix the salt and flour. Add the butter and pulse until it resembles chunky sand. Add the ice water and yogurt, pulse until everything is just combined. Add more water if needed to form a dough.

2. Lightly flour your surface and roll the dough into a rectangle to fit your baking sheet. Place the dough onto the sheet and chill for 30 minutes.

3. Set the oven to preheat at 400°F with the wire rack at the bottom of the oven.

4. When your dough is properly chilled, use a fork to poke holes all over the pastry and cover it with tin foil. Pour the uncooked rice over the foil. This will keep the pastry from puffing up too much. Place the sheet in the oven and bake for 20 minutes before removing the rice and foil and baking for an additional 5 minutes until the crust has browned. Put aside for later.

5. Whisk together the eggs and cream in a bowl and season with salt and pepper. Pour the egg mixture into the prepared crust and top with the asparagus. Place the sheet in the oven for 20-25 minutes until the filling is cooked and the crust is golden brown around the edges. Allow the tart to stand for 5 minutes before attempting to remove it from the sheet.

6. Cut and serve plain or with a side of your choice.

BUTTERNUT PIE

COOK TIME: 20 MINS | MAKES: 4 SERVING

INGREDIENTS:

- 2 tbsp. water
- 1 medium butternut, peeled and, cut into chunks
- olive cooking spray\olive oil
- 8 sheets pre-made puff pastry
- 1\2 cup parmesan cheese, shredded
- 1 cup canned pumpkin
- salt
- pepper
- 1\4 cup pecan nuts

- 1\4 cup sage leaves, torn
- 2 tbsp. melted butter
- 4 cups curly endive lettuce, shredded
- 2 tbsp. lemon juice

DIRECTIONS:

1. Set the oven to preheat at 450°F and line a baking sheet with greaseproof paper.

2. Place the butternut in a microwave-safe bowl with 2 tablespoons of water with the lid on. Toss the bowl to coat the butternut with water and microwave on high for 5 minutes or until the butternut is fork-tender. Discard excess water.

3. Use olive oil spray or normal olive oil between each layer of pastry as you layer them onto your prepared baking sheet.

4. In a large bowl, combine the parmesan with pumpkin, and 1\2 teaspoon each of salt and pepper.

5. Pour the pumpkin mixture onto the top layer of pastry and spread it around, leaving a 2-inch border on all sides. Top with the cooked squash, pecan nuts, and torn sage leaves. Pour the melted butter over the filling. Turn the edges over and pinch to form a border. Place the sheet in the oven and bake for 15-20 minutes or until the pie is nicely browned.

6. The pie can be served immediately with the endive salad tossed with lemon juice and a pinch of salt and pepper.

ROASTED HALLOUMI & VEG BARLEY

COOK TIME: 30 MINS | MAKES: 4 SERVINGS

INGREDIENTS:

- 1 cup rolled barley, rinsed, and drained
- olive oil
- 1 bay leaf
- 2 cups vegetable stock
- 2 delicata squash, peeled and cut into 1\2-inch slices
- 4 golden beets, peeled and cut into 1\4-inch slices
- 8 small cipollini onions, peeled
- 4 parsnips, peeled and cut into 1\4-inch strips

- pepper
- salt
- 4 sprigs thyme
- 3\4 lb. halloumi, cut into 1\2-inch cubes
- 1\4 cup tangy mayonnaise
- 2 tbsp. honey
- 2 tbsp. apple cider vinegar
- 2 tbsp. tahini
- 2 cups brussel sprout leaves, blanched

DIRECTIONS:

1. Set the oven to preheat at 425°F with 2 wire racks spaced evenly in the middle of the oven.

2. In a saucepan, heat the oil over medium heat and stir the barley for 1 minute after adding. Mix in the bay leaf and vegetable stock, allow the barley to simmer for 30 minutes or until all the water is gone and the barley is tender. Use a fork to separate the barley and set aside.

3. In a large bowl, combine the delicata squash, beets, onions, and parsnips with 2 tablespoons of olive oil and season with pepper and salt. Coat a baking sheet with a light layer of olive oil. Arrange the vegetables on the sheet and place the thyme sprigs on top. Bake in the oven for 10 minutes before removing the sheet from the oven and turning the vegetables with a spatula.

4. On a second lightly oiled baking sheet, place the Halloumi slices and use a basting brush to coat the tops. Return both sheets to the oven and bake for 5 minutes with the cheese on the lower rack. Turn the cheese after 5 minutes and bake for an additional 5 minutes on the other side. You can remove the vegetables if they are fork-tender. The cheese should be nicely toasted. Add the cooked barley to the vegetables and gently toss.

5. In a small bowl, beat the mayonnaise, honey, vinegar, and tahini. Season with salt and pepper to taste.

6. Divide the barley and vegetables between the plates, top with the cheese and Brussel sprout leaves. Drizzle with the sauce or serve on the side

VEGETARIAN PATTY SALAD

COOK TIME: 30 MINS | MAKES: 6 SERVINGS

INGREDIENTS:

- 1 cup fresh mint leaves
- 1 tsp. ground cumin
- 3 garlic cloves
- 1 tsp. crushed cilantro seeds
- 1 cup parsley, chopped
- 1 tsp. lemon zest
- himalayan salt
- black pepper
- 3 tbsp. all-purpose flour
- 15 Oz. chickpeas, rinsed, and drained
- 1\2 cup cold water

- 2 tbsp. olive oil
- 1\3 cup tahini sauce
- 1\2 shallot, finely chopped
- 1 lb. tomatoes, chopped
- 2 cucumbers, chopped
- 1\2 lemon, juiced
- toasted wraps for serving (optional)

DIRECTIONS:

1. Set the oven to preheat at 425°F and lightly coat a baking sheet with baking spray.

2. In a blender, pulse mint, cumin, garlic, cilantro seeds, 1\2 cup parsley, lemon zest, and 1\2 teaspoon each of salt and pepper until everything is combined. Add the flour and chickpeas to the blender and pulse until everything is properly mixed. You may need to stop and push some of the mixture back down so that everything is properly combined.

3. Roll the mixture into 12 balls of roughly the same size. Use a spatula or wooden spoon to press the balls down and form the patties. Arrange the patties on your prepared baking sheet and spray the tops with baking spray before placing the sheet in the oven and baking for 15 minutes. Flip the patties with a spatula and bake for an additional 10-15 minutes until the patties are browned on both sides.

4. In a glass bowl, beat the water, olive oil, and tahini to make the sauce.

5. In a separate bowl, combine 1\2 cup parsley, shallots, tomatoes, and cumber with the lemon juice and season with salt and pepper to taste.

6. Serve the patties on a bed of the salad and drizzle with the tahini sauce or fold into wraps.

ANGEL HAIR SOYBEAN PASTA

COOK TIME: 30 MINS | MAKES: 4-6 SERVINGS

INGREDIENTS:

- 2 tbsp. balsamic vinegar
- 2 tbsp. raw honey
- 2 tbsp. tamari
- 1 tsp. garlic powder
- 2 tbsp. vegetable oil
- 8 1\2 lb. frozen tempeh
- 1 yellow bell pepper, thinly sliced
- 1 red bell pepper, thinly sliced

- 2 carrots, cut julienne
- 1 shallot, thinly sliced
- 1 tbsp. vegetable oil
- 5 oz. angel hair pasta
- 1 cup baby soybeans, shelled
- 3 tbsp. tamari
- 1\2 cup coriander leaves, finely chopped

DIRECTIONS:

1. Set the oven to preheat at 425°F with the wire rack in the middle of the oven.

2. Whisk together the balsamic vinegar, raw honey, tamari, garlic powder, and vegetable oil. Add the tempeh and let it marinate for 5 minutes. Coat a baking sheet with baking spray. Arrange the coated tempeh on the sheet and bake for 5 minutes until browned. You can turn it halfway through if it starts to burn.

3. In the same bowl you used for the glaze, add the bell peppers, carrots, and shallot with the oil and toss to coat. Place the coated vegetables between the tempeh and return the sheet to the oven for 10 minutes.

4. In a large pot, cover the beans and pasta with water. Bring to a boil and remove from the heat. Let sit for 3 minutes until the pasta is soft before draining.

5. Toss the pasta and peas with the vegetables and tempeh. Plate and garnish with the extra tamari and coriander leaves if desired.

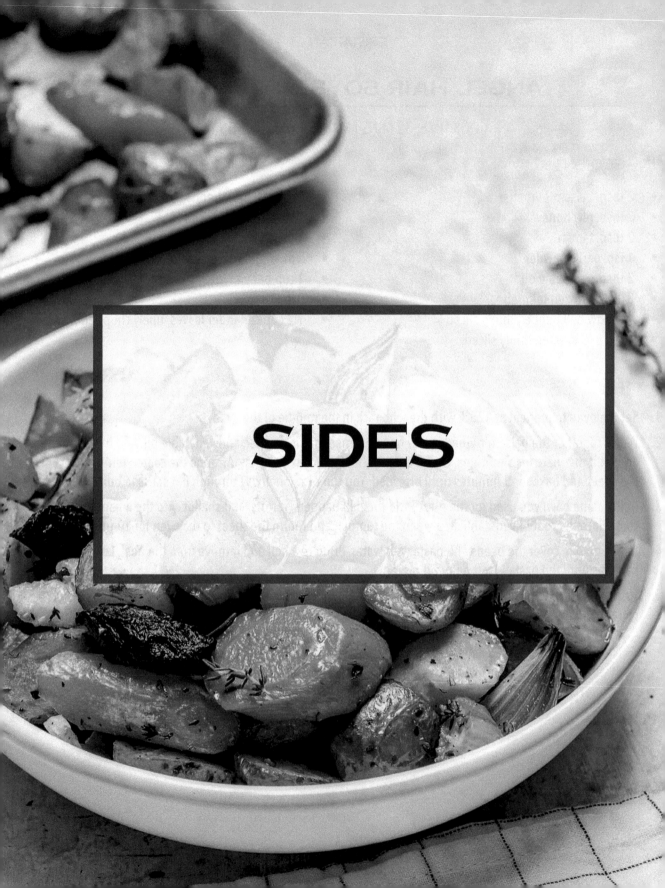

SIDES

YAM FRIES

COOK TIME: 50 MINS | MAKES: 4 SERVINGS

INGREDIENTS:

- 1\4 cup olive oil
- 1 3\4 lb. yams, peeled, and cut into fries
- 1\2 tsp. black pepper
- 1 tsp. himalayan salt
- 1 tbsp. fresh parsley, chopped
- 1\4 cup parmesan cheese, grated

DIRECTIONS:

1. Set the oven to preheat at 425°F and place a lightly sprayed baking sheet in the oven for 5 minutes while you prepare the fries.

2. In a large bowl, combine the oil, yam fries, pepper, and salt. Mix until evenly coated.

3. With oven gloves, remove the heated sheet from the oven, taking care not to burn. Place the fries on the sheet and return the sheet to the oven for 50 minutes. Flip the fries with a spatula whenever it looks like they are starting to brown. The fries are done when they are crispy.

4. Remove the fries from the oven and sprinkle with cheese and parsley to serve.

SMOKED-HAM WRAPPED ASPARAGUS PARCELS

COOK TIME: 12-15 MINS | MAKES: 4-6 SERVINGS

INGREDIENTS:

- olive oil
- 2 slices thinly cut smoked ham, cut into long strips
- 1 lb. asparagus, cleaned and trimmed
- black pepper
- himalayan salt
- 2 tbsp. fresh chives, finely chopped
- 2 tbsp. parmesan, grated.

DIRECTIONS:

1. Set the oven to preheat at 425°F and lightly coat a baking sheet with olive oil.

2. In a large bowl, toss together the cleaned asparagus, 1\2 teaspoon pepper, 1 teaspoon salt, chives, and 1 tablespoon olive oil until the asparagus is evenly coated.

3. Place your ham strips on the prepared sheet with 4-5 asparagus sticks at one end, wrap the ham around the asparagus bundle. Repeat with the remaining ham and asparagus. Sprinkle the parcels with cheese and bake in the oven for 12-15 minutes or until the asparagus is fork-tender.

SPICY ROASTED PEPPER SQUASH

COOK TIME: 40 MINS | MAKES: 6 SERVINGS

INGREDIENTS:

- 2 pepper squash
- black pepper
- himalayan salt
- 3 tbsp. olive oil
- 2 tsp. cayenne pepper
- 1 tsp. ground cumin
- 1\2 tsp. paprika

DIRECTIONS:

1. Set the oven to preheat at 400°F. Lightly coat a baking sheet with olive oil.

2. Halve the pepper squash and trim off the ends. Slice the halves into 1-inch rounds.

3. In a large bowl, toss the rounds with a pinch of salt and pepper, olive oil, cayenne pepper, cumin, and paprika. Arrange the rounds on the baking sheet and bake for 35-40 minutes, turning halfway through. The rounds are done when they are fork-tender and golden brown.

FANCY BRUSSELS SPROUTS

COOK TIME: 30 MINS | MAKES: 4 SERVINGS

INGREDIENTS:

- 1 small shallot, chopped
- 1 lb. brussels sprouts, trimmed and halved
- 1 tsp. salt
- 1\4 tsp. balck pepper
- 2 tbsp. olive oil
- 4 slices thick-cut bacon
- 1 tbsp. chives, chopped

DIRECTIONS:

1. Coat a baking sheet with baking spray and set the oven to preheat at 425°F.

2. In a bowl. Coat the shallots and Brussels sprouts with salt, pepper, and olive oil. Transfer the coated shallots and Brussels sprouts to the prepared baking sheet and fan them out. Bake in the oven for 15 minutes.

3. Meanwhile, cut the bacon into long slices. Remove the baking sheet from the oven after 15 minutes and mix the bacon strips with the Brussel sprouts before returning the sheet to the oven for an additional 15 minutes or until the bacon is crispy and the sprouts are tender.

SOUR CREAM & CHIVE SPUDS

COOK TIME: 65 MINS| MAKES: 4 SERVINGS

INGREDIENTS:

- 2 large potatoes
- olive oil
- 1\4 cup sour cream
- 1\4 cup greek yogurt, unsweetened
- 1\2 tsp. black pepper
- 1\2 tsp. salt
- 3 tbsp. fresh chives, chopped
- 1 cup grated mozzarella
- 1 green onion sliced
- 2 slices thick-cut bacon, cubed and cooked

DIRECTIONS:

1. Set the oven to preheat at 400°F.

2. Lightly coat a baking sheet with olive oil. Use a fork to poke small holes all over the potato. Use extra olive oil to rub a layer of oil all over the potatoes before placing them on the sheet and baking for 1 hour or until a knife can easily be inserted into a potato. Remove the sheet from the oven and allow the potatoes to cool.

3. Halve the potatoes and spoon the insides into a bowl. Try not to damage the skin. Leave the potato shells on the sheet. Add the sour cream, yogurt, pepper, salt, 1\2 cup mozzarella, and chives to the bowl. Mix until everything is just combined. Divide the mixture between the potato shells and top with the remaining mozzarella. Place the sheet in the oven for about 5 minutes until the cheese has just begun to melt.

4. Remove the sheet and set the oven to broil. Sprinkle the potatoes with bacon and spring onions before returning the sheet to the oven and broiling for 2-3 minutes until the cheese is nice and crispy.

ROASTED CAULIFLOWER WITH CAPERS

COOK TIME: 30 MINS | MAKES: 2-4 SERVINGS

INGREDIENTS:

- 1 large head of cauliflower
- olive oil
- 1\4 cup capers
- 4 anchovy filets in olive oil, chopped
- 3 tsp. crushed garlic
- black pepper

- salt
- 1 bunch spinach, chopped
- 1 bunch swiss chard, chopped
- 1\4 cup dried cherries
- 1\2 lemon juiced

DIRECTIONS:

1. Line a baking sheet with tinfoil and set the oven to preheat at 400°F.

2. Starting from the stem, slice the whole cauliflower into semi-thick rounds. If any pieces break off just place them next to the whole rounds on the baking sheet. Use a basting brush to coat both sides of your rounds with olive oil and arrange them on half of the baking sheet.

3. In a large bowl, combine the capers, anchovies, and garlic with 2 tablespoons of olive oil. Spoon the mixture in even amounts onto the cauliflower rounds and season with a pinch of salt and pepper. Place the sheet in the oven for 10 minutes or until the cauliflower is just starting to become tender. Remove the sheet from the oven.

4. In another bowl, Coat the spinach and Swiss chard with 3 tablespoons of olive oil and season with a pinch of salt and pepper. Spread the greens out on the other half of the sheet and bake for about 10 minutes before turning and baking for an additional 10 minutes until the greens have reduced in size and the cauliflower rounds are nicely toasted. They should be tender when poked with a fork.

5. Remove the sheet from the oven and drizzle the greens with the cherries and lemon juice. Serve on the side of the cauliflower rounds.

SEASONAL ROAST VEGETABLES

COOK TIME: 40 MINS | MAKES: 8 SERVINGS

INGREDIENTS:

- 8 cups of chopped mixed vegetables. (yams, butternut, turnips, and brussel sprouts.)
- 1 tbsp. salt
- 3 tbsp. olive oil
- 2 tbsp. raw honey
- 1 tbsp. soy sauce
- 3 tbsp. white miso
- 1\4 cup rice vinegar

- 2 tsp. sesame oil
- 3 spring onions, chopped
- 2 tbsp. toasted sesame seeds

DIRECTIONS:

1. Place two wire racks in the second slots from the top and bottom of the oven and set the oven to preheat at 400°F. Line a baking sheet with greaseproof paper.

2. Clean, trim and chop all of the vegetables. Place them in a bowl and coat with salt and olive oil. Spread the vegetables out over the baking sheet. You can use a second baking sheet if the vegetables do not fit on one sheet. If you use a second sheet, remember to alternate the sheets on the top and bottom racks for even cooking. Bake the vegetables for 30-40 minutes. They should be nicely browned and fork-tender. Remove the sheet or sheets from the oven and place the vegetables in a large bowl.

3. In a small bowl, beat the honey, soy sauce, miso, vinegar, and sesame oil. Drizzle the sauce over the vegetables and garnish with the spring onions and sesame seeds.

SPICY VEGETARIAN TOFU SKEWERS

COOK TIME: 30 MINS | MAKES: 4 SERVINGS

INGREDIENTS:

- 1 lb. tofu, extra firm
- 1\2 cup olive oil
- black pepper
- salt
- 1 1\2 tsp. ground cumin
- 2 lemons, juiced
- 16 cherry tomatoes
- 2 courgettes, cut into 1-inch pieces
- chinese yams, cut into 1-inch pieces
- 2 purple onions, halved lengthwise
- 2 poblano chilies, halved lengthwise
- 1 garlic clove
- 1\2 cup coriander leaves, chopped
- 1 lime, juiced
- 1\2 cup sour cream

DIRECTIONS:

1. Halve the tofu. You will need 6 paper towels, place the halved tofu on a plate in the middle of the paper towels, 3 underneath and 3 on top. Cover the tofu with another plate and use something heavy like a book to squash it down. Repeat after 5 minutes using new paper towels. Slice the tofu into 1-inch squares.

2. Line a baking sheet with tin foil and set the oven to preheat at 400°F.

3. Whisk together the olive oil, 1\2 teaspoon salt, 1\2 teaspoon pepper, cumin, and lemon juice in a bowl. Mix in the tofu, tomatoes, courgettes, and yams. Set aside on the counter for 15 minutes, stirring when half the time is done.

4. Build your skewers, alternating with the tofu and vegetables. Place your skewers on half the pan and the chilies and onions on the other half. Place the sheet in the oven for 15 minutes. After 15 minutes, remove the sheet from the oven and move the onions and chilies to a plate. Bake the skewers for an additional 10-12 minutes or until the vegetables are soft. Place the sheet on the counter and make a dome over the skewers using tin foil.

5. Transfer the chilies and onions to a blender and pulse with the garlic and coriander leaves. Push every-thing down using a wooden spoon before adding the lime juice and sour cream. Pulse until everything is properly combined as a sauce. Season to taste with salt and pepper.

6. Pour the sauce over the skewers or on the side as a dip.

(Quick Tip) If you are using wooden skewers, soak them in water for 30 minutes before use to stop them from burning.

MOZZARELLA CORN SALAD

COOK TIME: 25 MINS | MAKES: 4 SERVINGS

INGREDIENTS:

- olive oil
- 4 purple scallions, trimmed and chopped
- black pepper
- himalayan salt
- 4 corn ears, cleaned
- balsamic vinegar
- 1 lb. asparagus, trimmed
- 1 cup mozzarella, grated
- 3 radishes, cleaned and thinly sliced

DIRECTIONS:

1. Line a baking sheet with tin foil and set the oven to preheat at 425°F.

2. Coat the scallions with 3 tablespoons of olive oil and season with a pinch of salt and pepper. Use a basting brush to evenly coat the 4 ears of corn with 1 tablespoon of oil and season with salt and pepper to taste. Place the corn on one side of the baking sheet and the scallions on the other half. Bake in the oven for 15 minutes.

3. While the scallions and corn are roasting, coat the asparagus in a bowl with 1 tablespoon of olive oil and 2 teaspoons of vinegar. Add salt and pepper to taste.

4. After 15 minutes, remove the sheet from the oven and add the seasoned asparagus. Return the sheet to the oven and bake for an additional 10 minutes. All the vegetables should be soft when poked with a knife.

5. When the vegetables are done, remove the sheet from the oven and allow the vegetables to cool. Remove the corn kernels from the ear and toss them together with all the vegetables from the baking sheet.

6. In a separate bowl, mix the cheese with 2 tablespoons of oil and 2 teaspoons of vinegar. Plate the salad and top with the seasoned cheese. Use the radish slices as garnish.

ROASTED CHINESE AUBERGINES WITH TOFU

COOK TIME: 30 MINS | MAKES: 4 SERVINGS

INGREDIENTS:

- 14 oz. tofu, extra firm
- 1\4 tsp. cayenne pepper
- 2 tsp. crushed garlic
- 1 tsp. crushed ginger
- 2 tbsp. rice wine vinegar
- 2 tbsp. dark sesame oil
- 1\4 cup vegetable oil

- 1\3 cup soy sauce
- 1\2 lb. haricot verts, trimmed
- 3 chinese aubergines, cut into 1-inch pieces
- salt
- pepper

DIRECTIONS:

1. Halve the tofu. You will need 6 paper towels, place the halved tofu on a plate in the middle of the paper towels, 3 underneath and 3 on top. Cover the tofu with another plate and use something heavy like a book to squash it down. Repeat after 5 minutes using new paper towels. Slice the tofu into 3\4-inch squares.

2. Line a baking sheet with tin foil and set the oven to preheat at 400°F.

3. To make the marinade. Whisk together the cayenne pepper, garlic, ginger, vinegar, sesame oil, vegetable oil, and soy sauce. Add the tofu squares and toss the bowl until the tofu is evenly coated. Set aside on the counter and allow the marinade to sink in for about 20 minutes. You can stir the tofu more than once while it is marinating.

4. Arrange the vegetables on your prepared baking sheet alongside the tofu and season with salt and pepper. Place the sheet in the oven for 30 minutes, stirring after the first 15 minutes. The Tofu should be nice and crispy and the vegetables tender when poked with a fork.

FRENCH ROASTED BLISS POTATO SALAD

COOK TIME: 35 MINS | MAKES: 9 SERVINGS

INGREDIENTS:

- 2 tbsp. olive oil
- 2 lb. red bliss potatoes, quartered
- 1 tbsp. parsley, chopped
- 2 tbsp. chives, chopped
- 1\2 tsp salt
- 1\4 tsp. black pepper

- 1 tsp. french mustard
- 1 tsp. lemon juice
- 1 tbsp. onion powder
- 3 tbsp. white wine vinegar
- 1\3 cup sour cream

DIRECTIONS:

1. Set the oven to preheat at 400°F.

2. Use the olive oil to coat the potatoes before arranging them on a lightly oiled baking sheet. Place the sheet in the oven for 30-35 minutes until the potatoes are soft and just beginning to crisp.

3. In a large bowl, combine the parsley, chives, salt, pepper, mustard, lemon juice, onion powder, vinegar, and sour cream. Beat until everything is properly combined. Add the roast potatoes and coat. Serve immediately or store overnight in the fridge for a cold salad.

ROASTED HARICOT VERTS

COOK TIME: 25 MINS | MAKES: 4 SERVINGS

INGREDIENTS:

- 2 tsp. crushed garlic
- 10 oz. haricot verts, trimmed
- 1\2 tsp. black pepper

- 1\2 tsp. himalayan salt
- 1 tbsp. olive oil

DIRECTIONS:

1. Set the oven to preheat at 425°F.

2. Toss all the ingredients together in a large bowl, making sure that everything is evenly coated.

3. Spread the haricot verts out on a lightly oiled baking sheet and roast for 25 minutes in the bottom of the oven. Flip the beans with a spatula after 10 minutes.

CHEESY BEETROOT WITH NUTS

COOK TIME: 20 MINS | MAKES: 4 SERVINGS

INGREDIENTS:

- 3\4 lb. beetroot, cleaned, peeled, and sliced
- himalayan salt
- 2 tbsp. pecans, chopped
- 2 tbsp. fetta, crumbled

DIRECTIONS:

1. Lightly coat a baking sheet with baking spray and set the oven to preheat at 400°F.

2. Layer the beetroot slices on the prepared baking sheet and, it's okay if some slices overlap, sprinkle with a pinch of salt and bake in the oven for 18-20 minutes.

3. Plate the beets and garnish with the nuts and cheese.

SWISS-CHEESE GARLIC LOAF

COOK TIME: 2 MINS | MAKES: 1 LOAF, 12 SLICES

INGREDIENTS:

- 1 (9 oz.) french breadstick
- 1 1\2 tbsp. olive oil vinaigrette
- 2 tsp. crushed garlic
- 1\2 cup swiss asiago cheese, grated
- 1\2 tsp. rosemary, chopped

DIRECTIONS:

1. Line a baking sheet with tin foil and preheat the broiler.

2. Place the French breadstick on the pan and make 12 diagonal slices across the loaf.

3. In a small bowl, whisk together the vinegar and crushed garlic. Use a basting brush to coat the loaf with the vinegar mixture, make sure you get between the slices as well.

4. Push the cheese between the slices and sprinkle some on top of the loaf. Top with the rosemary. Place the sheet in the oven until the cheese is melted. This should only take about 2 minutes. Serve straight away.

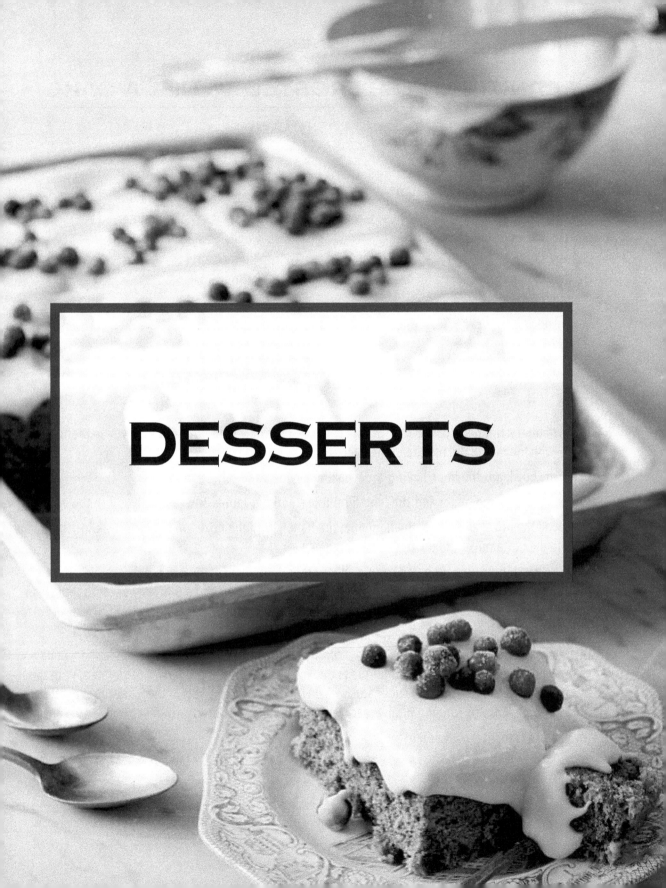

DESSERTS

PEANUT BUTTER FROSTED VANILLA CAKE

COOK TIME: 17 MINS | MAKES: 1 CAKE

INGREDIENTS:

- 3 cups cake flour (extra for the sheet)
- 1 tbsp. baking soda
- 3\4 tsp baking powder
- 3\4 tsp. salt
- 16 tbsp. butter, cubed (extra for the sheet)
- 1 cup brown sugar
- 1 1\2 tsp. vanilla essence
- 3 large eggs
- 1 1\2 cups buttermilk

- 5 tbsp. butter, room temperature
- 1 1\2 cups smooth peanut butter
- 1 tbsp. vanilla essence
- 1\2 cup light cream
- 4-5 cups icing sugar

DIRECTIONS:

1. Lightly butter a rimmed 13 x 18-inch baking sheet and sprinkle with flour. Set the oven to preheat at 350°F with the rack in the middle of the oven.

2. In a large bowl, mix the flour, baking soda, baking powder, and salt. Set aside

3. In a mixer, cream the butter and sugar for 5 minutes. Add the vanilla and gradually mix in the eggs.

4. Switch off the mixer and empty the flout onto the batter. With the mixer on the lowest setting, gradually work in the buttermilk until the batter is lump-free.

5. Pour the batter onto your prepared baking sheet, smoothing it out with an offset spatula. Place the sheet in the oven and bake for 15-17 minutes or until the top is browned and a thin skewer comes out clean when inserted in the middle. Remove the sheet from the oven and allow the cake to completely cool for about 2 hours on the sheet.

6. In a clean bowl, use the mixer on medium to combine the butter and peanut butter. Add the vanilla and cream while the mixer is running. Continue to mix until everything is properly incorporated. With the mixer off, add 3 cups of the icing sugar and beat on medium. Add the rest of the icing sugar a little at a time while the mixer is running until it reaches the desired consistency.

7. Ice the cake when it is completely cool.

TOASTED PECAN MARSHMALLOW CAKE

COOK TIME: 40 MINS | MAKES: 15 SERVINGS

INGREDIENTS:

- 1 cup pecans, chopped
- 4 oz. milk chocolate, chopped
- 16 tbsp. butter
- 1 1\2 cups all-purpose flour
- 2 cups white sugar
- 1\2 cup cocoa powder
- 3\4 tsp. salt
- 1 tsp. vanilla essence

- 4 large eggs
- 10 1\2 0z. miniature marshmallows
- frosting:
- 8 tbsp. butter
- 1\3 cup milk
- 1\3 cup cocoa powder
- 1 tsp. vanilla essence
- 16 oz. icing sugar

DIRECTIONS:

1. Set the oven to preheat at 350°F. Lightly butter and flour a baking sheet that has a 1-inch high rim.

2. Spread the pecans out over a large baking sheet and scorch them in the oven for 8-10 minutes.

3. Place the chocolate and 1 cup of butter in a glass bowl and microwave on high for 1 minute, stirring after 30 seconds until everything is melted.

4. In a separate bowl, combine the flour, sugar, cocoa powder, and salt with a whisk. Beat in the vanilla and eggs. Whisk in the chocolate and butter mixture to form a lump-free batter. Pour the batter into your prepared sheet and bake in the middle of the oven for 20 minutes. Remove the sheet from the oven and spread the mini marshmallows over the cake before returning the sheet to the oven and baking for an additional 8-10 minutes or until the marshmallows have browned, campfire-style.

5. In a clean glass bowl, melt the 8 tablespoons of butter on high for 30 seconds. Beat in the milk and cocoa powder until the mixture begins to thicken. Use a handheld mixer to incorporate the vanilla and icing sugar until everything is lump-free and properly combined.

6. Ice the warm cake immediately and decorate the icing with the scorched pecans.

RUBY-TOPPED OREO CHEESECAKE

COOK TIME: 35 MINS | MAKES: 1 CAKE

INGREDIENTS:

- 10 tbsp. butter
- 1 family-sized bagged oreos
- 1 cup ricotta cheese
- 1 3\4 cups caster sugar
- 1 3\4 cups cream cheese
- 4 1\2 tsp. vanilla essence
- 6 large eggs
- 5 tbsp. cake flour
- 1 1\4 cup seedless raspberry jam

DIRECTIONS:

1. Set the oven to preheat at 325°F with the wire rack in the middle of the oven.

2. In a blender, crumb the cookies a few at a time until they are all in and the mixture resembles coarse sand. In a large bowl, melt the butter in the microwave, add the Oreo sand to the melted butter and mix with a wooden spoon.

3. Spoon the mixture onto a 13 x 18-inch rimmed baking sheet and use clean hands or the bottom of a glass to press the crust evenly onto the sheet and up the sides.

4. Using a mixer, beat the ricotta, caster sugar, and cream cheese for about 4 minutes until the mixture is light and fluffy. Beat in the vanilla and gradually add the eggs. Finally, beat in the flour until there are no lumps and everything is properly combined. Pour the batter onto the crust and bake in the oven for 35 minutes until the center is firm and the top is golden. Remove the sheet from the oven and allow the cake to cool for about 3 hours before transferring it to the fridge and chilling overnight.

5. When the cake is properly chilled the following day, place your raspberry jam in a glass bowl and micro-wave for about 10 seconds. Whisk the jam until it is smooth. If the jam is hot, allow it to cool for a few minutes before spreading it on your cheesecake with an offset spatula.

CHOCOLATE CHIP PEANUT BUTTER SQUARES

COOK TIME: 20 MINS | MAKES: 24 SQUARES

INGREDIENTS:

- 1 tsp. vanilla essence
- 2 large eggs
- 3\4 cup chunky peanut butter
- 2 cups bisquick
- 1 cup dark brown sugar
- 12 oz. chocolate chips

DIRECTIONS:

1. Set the oven to preheat at 325°F. Lightly spray a rimmed baking sheet with baking spray.

2. Use a wooden spoon to beat the vanilla, eggs, and peanut butter. Add the Bisquick, sugar, and 3\4 cups of the chocolate chips and mix until everything is just combined. Do not over mix.

3. Transfer the batter to your prepared baking sheet and use an offset spatula to spread it out, you can use your hands if the batter is too thick.

4. Place the sheet in the oven for about 20 minutes or until the batter is nicely browned. Remove the sheet from the oven and drizzle immediately with the rest of the chocolate chips. Allow all the chips to melt, then take a clean spatula and spread the chocolate out.

5. Cut into squares and serve with a dollop of ice cream or store in an airtight container for later.

SWIRLED PRETZEL BRICKLE WITH PEANUTS

COOK TIME: 10 MINS | MAKES: 1 SHEET

INGREDIENTS:

- 8 oz. white baking chocolate, finely chopped
- 8 oz. brown baking chocolate, finely chopped
- 1\2 cup crushed pretzels
- 1\2 cup roasted peanuts

DIRECTIONS:

1. Set the oven to preheat at 200°F and line a small baking sheet with greaseproof paper, allowing the sides to extend beyond the sheet about 2-inches.

2. Toss the two kinds of chocolate together on the baking sheet. Turn off the oven before placing the sheet in the oven for about 10 minutes or until all the chocolate has melted.

3. Use the tip of a skewer to make swirls in the chocolate layer before sprinkling the pretzels and peanuts over the chocolate. Place the sheet in the fridge for about 30 minutes or until the chocolate has set.

4. Grip the edges of the paper and pull the brickle out of the sheet. Brake or cut into rough pieces.

SALTED CARAMEL PRETZEL CAKE

COOK TIME: 20 MINS | MAKES: 1 SHEET CAKE

INGREDIENTS:

- 6 tbsp. cocoa powder
- 1 cup warm water
- 2 1\4 cups all-purpose flour, plus 2 tbsp.
- 1\2 tsp. salt
- 1 1\4 tsp. baking soda
- 19 tbsp. butter, cubed
- 1 cup white sugar
- 1 cup dark brown sugar
- 1 egg white
- 2 large eggs

- 1 tbsp. vanilla essence
- 1\2 cup sour cream
- for the frosting:
- 1\4 cup butterscotch caramel sauce
- 19 tbsp. butter, room temperature
- 1 1\2 tsp. vanilla essence
- 1\3 cup sour cream
- 2-3 cups icing sugar
- 3 cups mini pretzels (or crushed regular pretzels)

DIRECTIONS:

1. Set the oven to preheat at 350°F with the wire rack in the middle of the oven. Butter and flour a 13 x 18-inch rimmed baking sheet.

2. In a bowl, beat the cocoa powder into the warm water until all the lumps are gone. Let the mixture rest on the counter.

3. In a separate bowl, combine the flour, salt, and baking powder. Set aside.

4. Place the butter and all the sugar in a clean bowl and beat until light and fluffy. This should take approximately 5 minutes. Gradually add the egg white followed by the eggs while the mixer is running. You may want to stop and push all the batter down before you add the vanilla and sour cream. Once the batter is nice and smooth with the added vanilla and sour cream, gradually add the flour and cocoa mixtures, alternating between the two, until everything is added and you have a lump-free batter.

5. Pour the batter into your prepared sheet in an even layer. Place the sheet in the oven and bake for 18-20 minutes or until an inserted skewer comes out clean. Remove the sheet from the oven and allow the cake to cool in the sheet for about 2 hours.

6. For the frosting, beat 3\4 cups of the butterscotch caramel sauce with the butter for approximately 2 minutes before adding the vanilla and sour cream. Beat until everything is properly combined.

7. Gradually add the icing sugar, 1 cup at a time until it reaches the desired spreading consistency. Ice your cake with the frosting. You can decorate immediately or allow the icing to set a bit before you decorate with the pretzels. Pour the remaining butterscotch caramel sauce over the pretzels.

COCONUTTY JAM-POCKET CAKE

COOK TIME: 25 MINS | MAKES: 1 SHEET CAKE

INGREDIENTS:

- 4 ²\3 cups all-purpose flour
- 1 ½ tsp. baking powder
- ¼ tsp. salt
- 32 tbsp. butter, cubed
- 1 ¹\3 cups white sugar
- 1 tsp. vanilla essence
- 1 egg white

- 2 large eggs
- 2 ½ cup grated coconut
- 1 ½ cups jam of your preference

DIRECTIONS:

1. Set the oven to preheat at 350°F with the wire rack in the middle of the oven. Grease a 13 x 18-inch rimmed baking sheet.

2. In a large bowl, combine the flour, baking powder, and salt with a whisk.

3. Use a mixer to beat the butter, sugar, and vanilla for approximately 5 minutes until light and fluffy. Gradually beat in the egg white, followed by the eggs until your mixture is properly combined. Use a wooden spoon to mix in the flour mixture. You may want to use clean hands to form the dough as the mixture is thick.

4. Once you have a uniform dough. Use clean hands or the bottom of a glass to press the dough into the prepared sheet.

5. Drizzle the coconut evenly over the cake and use the bottom of your glass to press it into your dough.

6. Use the back of a teaspoon to press small pockets into your cake dough, about 80. Fill each pocket with a drop of jam, you don't want to overfill the pockets.

7. Place your sheet in the oven and bake for approximately 25 minutes until golden. Remove the cake from the oven and allow the cake to cool on the sheet before slicing and serving.

WALNUT-GLAZED APPLE SPONGE

COOK TIME: 30 MINS | MAKES: 1 SHEET

INGREDIENTS:

- 1 ³\4 cups brown sugar
- 7 granny smith apples, peeled, cored, and sliced
- 3 ²\3 cups all-purpose flour
- 1 tsp. ground cinnamon
- ½ tsp. nutmeg
- 1 ¼ tsp. baking powder

- ½ tsp. baking soda
- ½ tsp. salt
- 1 egg white
- 2 large eggs
- 2 tsp. vanilla essence
- ³\4 cups walnut oil
- 3 cups crushed walnuts

For the glaze:
- 3 tbsp. corn syrup
- 9 tbsp. water
- 1 tbsp. vanilla essence
- 4-5 cups icing sugar

DIRECTIONS:

1. In a large bowl, coat the apple slices with the sugar. Set the bowl aside for 30 minutes, allowing the apples to marinate in the sugar.

2. Set the oven to preheat at 350°F with the wire rack in the middle of the oven. Butter a 13 x 18-inch rimmed baking sheet.

3. In a medium bowl, combine the flour, cinnamon, nutmeg, baking powder, baking soda, and salt.

4. In the bowl with your marinated apple slices, mix in the egg white, 2 eggs, and vanilla. Add the walnut oil and mix until everything is properly combined. Add the flour mixture to the apples and mix until there are no lumps, but do not over mix.

5. Pour the mixture into your prepared sheet in an even layer. Bake in the oven for 25 minutes or until an inserted skewer comes out clean. Remove the sheet from the oven and allow the sponge to cool completely on the sheet.

6. While your sponge cools and the oven is still hot, spread your crushed walnuts over a baking sheet and scorch in the oven for about 6 minutes. You can flip them with a spatula if they start to burn. Remove the sheet from the oven and allow the walnuts to cool.

7. In a saucepan over medium heat, bring the water and corn syrup to a boil. Simmer for 1 minute before removing the mixture from the heat and adding the vanilla essence. Gradually stir in the icing sugar 1 cup at a time. You want a sloppy icing that can be poured.

8. Pour the warm glaze over the sponge, spreading it around with an offset spatula. Top with the scorched nuts.

9. You want to eat this sponge in one day as the apples will continue to soften over time.

FROSTED STRAWBERRY SPONGE

COOK TIME: 30 MINS | MAKES: 1 SHEET

INGREDIENTS:

- 2 ½ cups white sugar
- 20 tbsp. butter
- 5 large eggs
- 1 ½ tsp. vanilla essence
- 1 tbsp. lemon juice
- 1 tsp. salt
- 1 tsp. baking soda

- 3 oz. strawberry gelatin
- 3 cups all-purpose flour
- 1 ¼ cups buttermilk
- 1 cup strawberries, chopped
- 12 oz. ready-made vanilla frosting
- 1 cup fresh strawberries, halved

DIRECTIONS:

1. Set the oven to preheat at 350°F and line a medium-sized, rimmed baking sheet with greaseproof paper. Coat the greaseproof paper with a thin layer of baking spray.

2. Use a hand mixer to cream the sugar and butter until it's light and fluffy. Gradually add the eggs while the mixer is running. Add the vanilla and lemon juice.

3. In a separate bowl, whisk together the salt, baking soda, gelatin, and flour.

4. Begin adding the flour and buttermilk to the creamed butter while the mixer is on the lowest setting. Alternating between the two until everything is combined. Beat until the batter is lump-free. Finally, mix in the chopped strawberries.

5. Pour the batter into your prepared baking sheet in an even layer. Bake in the oven for approximately 30 minutes or until the top is golden and an inserted skewer comes out clean.

6. Allow the cake to cool completely on the baking sheet before frosting and decorating with the halved strawberries.

LEMON SPONGE WITH CURD FROSTING

COOK TIME: 30 MINS | MAKES: 1 SHEET

INGREDIENTS:

- 1\2 cup lemon juice
- 1\2 white sugar
- 6 tbsp. butter
- 3 large eggs

For the sponge:
- 3 cups all-purpose flour
- 1\2 tsp. salt
- 1\2 tsp. baking soda
- 9 tbsp. butter, cubed
- 1 1\2 cups brown sugar

- 1 tbsp. lemon zest
- 3 large eggs
- 3 egg whites
- 2 tsp. lemon essence
- 2 tsp. vanilla essence
- 5 tbsp. lemonade concentrate

For the frosting:
- 3\4 cup icing sugar
- 1\4 tsp. salt
- 1 1\2 cup heavy cream

DIRECTIONS:

1. Fit a glass bowl over a saucepan of simmering water. Place the lemon juice and sugar in the bowl and whisk the mixture until it's frothy. This should only take a few seconds. Beat in the butter, eggs, and lemon zest. Continually whisk the curd for approximately 12 minutes, until it starts to thicken. Chill the curd for a minimum of 4 hours or overnight before using.

2. Set the oven to preheat at 350°F with the wire rack in the middle of the oven. Butter a 13 x 18-inch rimmed baking sheet.

3. Whisk together the flour, salt, and baking soda. Set aside.

4. Cream the butter, sugar, and lemon zest with a mixer until light and fluffy. Turn off the mixer and push all the butter down, using a wooden spoon. Turn the mixer on again and gradually beat in the egg whites, followed by the eggs. Finally. Add the lemon essence, vanilla essence, and lemonade concentrate.

5. Turn the mixer off and mix the flour in with a wooden spoon, scraping the sides as you go. Turn the mixer back on and beat the batter until it is lump-free.

6. Pour the batter in an even layer onto your prepared baking sheet. Bake in the oven for 18-20 minutes or until the top is golden and an inserted skewer comes out clean. Allow the cake to cool on the sheet for a few hours.

7. Whisk together the icing sugar, salt, and heavy cream to form soft peaks. Gently fold in the chilled curd.

8. Ice the cake with the curd frosting.

NUTTY SPICED POKE CAKE

COOK TIME: 30 MINS | MAKES: 1 SHEET

INGREDIENTS:

- 3 ½ cups walnut pieces, chopped
- ½ tsp. salt
- ½ tsp. nutmeg
- 1 tsp. baking soda
- 1 tsp. ground cloves
- 1 ½ tsp. ground cinnamon
- 4 ½ tsp. baking powder
- 4 cups all-purpose flour

- 1 ½ cups white sugar
- 4 large eggs
- 1 $^1\backslash3$ cups plain yogurt
- 2 cups orange juice
- 1 tbsp. orange zest
- ½ cup sunflower oil
- 3 tbsp. butter
- $^3\backslash4$ cups dark brown sugar

DIRECTIONS:

1. Set the oven to preheat at 350°F with the wire rack in the middle of the oven. Butter a 13 x 18-inch rimmed baking sheet.

2. Use a second baking sheet to scorch the nuts in the oven for approximately 10 minutes. You can flip them with a spatula if they start to burn. Remove the sheet from the oven and set aside for later.

3. In a large bowl, combine salt, nutmeg, baking soda, cloves, cinnamon, baking powder, and flour.

4. Remove 1 1\2 cups of the walnuts and set aside. Pulse the rest of the walnuts in a food processor until finely chopped.

5. Beat the brown sugar and eggs with a mixer until light and fluffy. Beat in the yogurt. Add 1 cup of the orange juice, zest, and sunflower oil while the mixer is running. Turn off the mixer and use a wooden spoon to mix in the walnuts from the food processor and the flour mixture. Mix until the batter is lump-free.

6. Pour the batter onto your prepared baking sheet in an even layer. Place the sheet in the oven and bake for 20-25 minutes until an inserted skewer comes out clean.

7. Meanwhile, place 1 cup orange juice, 3 tablespoons butter, and 3\4 cups dark brown sugar in a saucepan. Stir the mixture over a high heat until all the granules disappear. Allow the mixture to thicken over the heat for approximately 6 minutes.

8. Once your cake is done. Use a chopstick to poke holes all over the cake. The more the merrier. Pour your hot syrup over the cake and decorate with the chopped walnuts.

CINNAMON CRUMBLED COFFEE SPONGE

COOK TIME: 38 MINS | MAKES: 1 SHEET

INGREDIENTS:

For the crumble:
- 1\2 tsp. Salt
- 2 tbsp. ground cinnamon
- 1 1\3 cups brown sugar
- 3 cups all-purpose flour
- 1 tbsp. Vanilla essence
- 16 tbsp. Butter, softened but not hot

For the cake:
- 1\2 tsp. Baking soda
- 1 tsp. Salt

- 1 1\4 tsp. Baking powder
- 4 3\4 cups all-purpose flour
- 19 tbsp. Butter, cubed
- 1 2\3 cups white sugar
- 2\3 cups dark brown sugar
- 1 egg yolk
- 3 large eggs
- 4 1\2 tsp. Vanilla essence
- 1 3\4 cups sour cream, plus 1 tbsp.

DIRECTIONS:

1. In a bowl, combine all the dry ingredients for the crumble. Add the vanilla and softened butter. With clean hands, work the mixture between your fingers until it resembles breadcrumbs, leaving a few bigger pieces for the texture. You don't want it too fine. Set aside for later.

2. Set the oven to preheat at 325°F with the wire rack in the middle of the oven. Use butter to grease a 13 x 18-inch rimmed baking sheet.

3. In a medium bowl, combine the baking soda, salt, baking powder, and flour. Set aside.

4. Cream the butter and 2 kinds of sugar in a mixer until light and fluffy. Gradually add the egg yolk, and the eggs while the mixer is running. Use a wooden spoon to push the mixture down before beating in the vanilla and sour cream. The batter should be lump-free. Turn the mixer off and use a wooden spoon to stir in the flour. It will be very thick.

5. Pour your batter onto the prepared baking sheet in an even layer. Sprinkle the crumble evenly over the batter.

6. Place the sheet in the oven and bake for 35-38 minutes or until an inserted skewer comes out clean. Remove the sheet from the oven and allow the sponge to cool before serving.

CRANBERRY SHEET SPONGE

COOK TIME: 35 MINS | MAKES: 1 SHEET

INGREDIENTS:

- 2 1\2 cups all-purpose flour
- 2 1\2 cups brown sugar
- 1 tap. baking powder
- 1\2 tsp. salt
- 20 tbsp. butter
- 5 large eggs
- 2 tsp. vanilla essence
- 1 1\2 cups chopped pecans
- 5 cups cranberries

DIRECTIONS:

1. Set the oven to preheat at 325°F with the wire rack in the middle of the oven. Use butter to grease a 13 x 18-inch rimmed baking sheet.

2. In a bowl, use a whisk to combine the flour, sugar, baking powder, and salt.

3. In a separate bowl, beat the butter, eggs, and vanilla. Pout this mixture into the flour and mix using a wooden spoon to form a thick batter. Stir in the pecans and cranberries.

4. Pour the batter into an even layer on the prepared sheet. Place the sheet in the oven and bake for 30-35 minutes or until an inserted skewer comes out clean. Remove the sheet from the oven and allow the cake to cool completely on the sheet before serving. Or serve hot with a scoop of ice cream.

CONCLUSION

I would like to personally thank every single one of you that has purchased this book.

It is an immense pleasure to not only gain this knowledge but share it with the world. By making cooking simpler and more enjoyable, we are not only encouraging healthier eating, but we are helping the world by discovering more ways to use energy more efficiently.

I hope you try each and every one of these recipes and adjust them to your specific tastes. My goal at the end of the day is that you have fun with your family and friends while enjoying simpler cooking techniques!

METRIC EQUIVALENCE CHART

Volume Measurements		Weight Measurements		Temperature Conversion	
U.S.	**Metric**	**U.S.**	**Metric**	**Fahrenheit**	**Celsius**
1 teaspoon	5 ml	1/2 ounce	15 g	250	120
1 tablespoon	15 ml	1 ounce	30 g	300	150
1/4 cup	60 ml	3 ounces	85 g	325	160
1/3 cup	80 ml	4 ounces	115 g	350	175
1/2 cup	125 ml	8 ounces	225 g	375	190
2/3 cup	160 ml	12 ounces	340 g	400	200
3/4 cup	180 ml	1 pound	450 g	425	220
1 cup	250 ml	2-1/4 pounds	1 kg	450	230